Plastic Surgery Tales:
A Look Behind the Face of the Specialty

by

Robert N. Cooper, M.D., P.A.

W.I.T. Book Publisher, Inc.   Stuart, Florida

Published by W.I.T. Book Publisher, Inc.
1352 SE Madison Avenue
Stuart, Florida 34996

Manufactured in the United States of America.

Library of Congress Control Numbers: 2001012345

ISBN: 1-892697-06-8

CONTENTS

Chapter IV Chance (continued)

Chapter V Physician As Doctor –
Doing One's Job

Chapter VI Empowerment

Chapter VII Humorous

Chapter VII Humorous (continued)

Chapter VIII The Human Condition

Chapter IX Recognition of a Job Well Done

Chapter X Self-Reliance

Dedication

When we encounter a natural style, we are always
surprised and delighted, for we thought to see an
author and found a man.
–Pascal

No single work shaped my thinking as a plastic surgeon more than did *The Patient and the Plastic Surgeon* by Dr. Robert Goldwyn. It provided more than handy tips; it taught me how to approach certain patient issues in a new way. For that I will be forever grateful.

Through his writings in our joural, *Plastic and Reconstructive Surgery*, Dr. Goldwyn has taught thousands of plastic surgeons how, not only to address difficult problems, but also how to view ourselves. Rapier wit tempered with a heaping dose of self-deprecation proved invaluable in debunking the silliness that seems to creep into many serious endeavors.

Topics covered the entire spectrum of the specialty. Controversial issues like "whether you are an Inny or an Outty" (about where on the ear the facelift incision would be placed) were put in proper perspective, relative to the quality of the surgery. Years ago he dealt with the internal marketing options by telling us of surgeons who inform their patients that silk imported from remote provinces in China makes the difference in the quality of their suturing. Some of the editorials were so funny they were passed around the office for all to enjoy.

But running through each editorial was a valuable pearl of wisdom. Much like the parable related by the clergyman during a sermon, there was truth and wisdom to be gleaned from within the story. The fact that the vast majority of the editorials were hysterically funny made the reading that much more enjoyable.

In an effort to thank Dr. Goldwyn for his many contributions, I contacted several hundred plastic surgeons around the world and asked if they would help honor him with their best stories. Each contributor related anecdotes understanding that a compilation of the stories would be collected as a tribute to Dr. Goldwyn.

I am humbled by the thought that the book that resulted from that effort is dwarfed by the works of Dr. Goldwyn. We, the contributors, thank you and dedicate this book to you, Dr. Goldwyn.

Robert N. Cooper, M.D., P.A.
Stuart, Florida

Acknowledgments

I would like to thank every plastic surgeon who contributed to this book. In some cases great effort was expended in sending me an edited, typewritten copy of the anecdote.

Many thanks to Lieutenant Commander John Lea and my wife, Mary, for the fine job of editing stories that were transcribed from tapes made often by surgeons for whom English is a second or third language. John, a former Royal Navy submarine commander, has written widely. He offers great wisdom as well as the critical ear of the layperson not steeped in medical jargon. Mary is a successful screenwriter with a substantial body of work as a comedy writer.

I would also like to thank Barbara Jean Hope a professional editor with W.I.T. Book Publisher, Inc., and Charles A. Powell, the publisher, for their commitment to making sure the book met the good standards of the American book industry.

Robert N. Cooper, M.D., P.A.
Stuart, Florida

Foreword

The true-life experiences of plastic surgeons offer far better tales than the fictional accounts related on shows like "Nip & Tuck" or the quasi reality of "Extreme Makeovers." The human side of the specialty has nothing to do with $4,500.00 suits or Ferraris. Every professional who has practiced for several years has had contact with enough people to generate some interesting if not wholly believable real-life tales of the human condition. I, too, had some anecdotes from my practice and training that in the great conceit of naivety I thought might be of interest to others.

It occurred to me several years ago that if I had some good stories, perhaps my colleagues would also have some interesting anecdotes. It was in that spirit that in early 2001 I started contacting hundreds of plastic surgeons all over the world and asked for their best stories. The goal was to collect an anthology of these anecdotes and dedicate the resulting book to Dr. Robert Goldwyn, the editor of our "Plastic and Reconstructive Surgery" journal. Please see this book's dedication.

Anecdotes, stories, and related tales came streaming in on tapes for the most part. These were then transcribed and edited. Every contributor was aware that the resulting book was undertaken to honor Dr. Goldwyn. In the event that any proceeds were generated from the project, those funds would be given to the Plastic Surgery Education Foundation. I wanted nothing but the stories.

Things were put on hold after September 11, 2001. I then got involved with an entry in the World Trade Center Memorial competition. I pressed on with the book and enjoyed a truly rewarding experience with the publisher.

This book is therefore an evocation of what the profession is and what it does. Chapters seemed appropriate, in their division of stories, as dramatic, tragic, unbelievable, humorous, unexpected or characteristic of the indomitable human spirit.

Robert N. Cooper, M.D.
Stuart, Florida

Chapter I

Misunderstandings

LOVE IS BLIND

BARRY ZIDE, M.D.   New York, NY

Mistakes are the portals of discovery.
—James Joyce

It must have been some fifteen years ago that a ten-year-old boy was brought by his parents for me to excise a solitary tumor on the front of his leg. It looked to be a simple enough procedure and, from a surgeon's viewpoint, not particularly interesting.

Much more interesting were the New York Jewish parents. The wife was some five-feet-eight-inches tall, brunette, stunning figure, absolutely beautiful. In a word, drop-dead gorgeous. The husband, on the other hand, was short, curly-haired, dumpy, quite ordinary looking.

The first thought that leapt into my mind when I met them was, "How did this guy ever end up with this incredibly beautiful woman?" I was amazed that they were together. They seemed like the perfect definition of a mismatch.

I recovered my train of thought and addressed them.

"Which one of you, Mr. and Mrs. . . ., would like to be with your son while I remove this from his leg?"

The boy's mother replied.

"We are no longer married, we're divorced."

Again my thoughts silently broke in on my professionalism. "Whew, I can understand that . . . I mean, God...this is the most unusual thing . . . what does this guy have, after all? is he rich? . . . the world's greatest lover?" It seemed completely appropriate that they were divorced because of the woman's astounding attractiveness – she just didn't seem like the sort of woman who would remain tied to this man.

She spoke again. "I'll stay with my son."

We went into the room behind my office. I got the local anesthetic out, and was just about to inject the boy's leg when the mother spoke.

"Dr. Zide, before you do that, I'd like you to say a chant."

I replied, "Oh, come on . . . be serious, now."

But she insisted.

"No, Dr. Zide, you may not inject my son's leg unless you do this chant." And for the next minute she chanted: "Ah booh galla, rum das, blah, blah, blah . . ."

I had to repeat every every word that she said for about two verses before I was allowed to make the injection.

The neurofibroma came out with no difficulty. I left the mother with her son and walked out to the ex-husband.

"You know, your former wife had me say a chant over your son before I injected the local anesthetic."

"Why do you think I left that crazy bitch?" he said.

A paradigm shift, indeed. I had jumped to entirely the wrong conclusion.

A NEW TUNE

BRUCE ACHAUER, M.D.　　　ORANGE, CA

A shlemiehl lands on his back and bruises his nose.
　　　　　　–Yiddish Proverb

A very pleasant lady in her mid-'60s elected to undergo her first rejuvenation surgery and chose procedures of the face and neck. In addition to a facelift and mid-face lift, she decided to undergo a chin advancement to correct a very retrusive chin. She had an excellent result and, after a few weeks' recovery, she felt well enough to sing in the choir and attend choir practice at her church. She was surprised to be approached by a single gentleman of her own age who overwhelmed her with attention, compliments, and helpful hints about the choir.

"So," he said, "are you new to this church?"

"Not really," she replied. "I've been singing in the choir with you for the past 12 years."

ARTISTRY

BRUNNO RISTOW, M.D.
SAN FRANCISCO, CA

I have an instinct for loving the truth;
but only an instinct.
—Voltaire

I call it the "love is blind" phenomenon.

Feedback from patients who have undergone cosmetic plastic surgery report that their nearest and dearest are aware that their appearance has become more youthful, more attractive, but do not necessarily attribute it to surgery. Let me give you an example.

A recently retired school teacher underwent a face and neck lift, a forehead lift, eyelid lift, and correction of a prominent nose. I had forewarned her that the results would be striking. On the tenth day after surgery, I put a key question to her: "How does your husband like the result?"

"Oh," she replied, "I haven't told him. He is away in Europe for four weeks on business."

When she returned for her one-month follow-up, I asked again about her husband's reaction.

"Well, the moment I opened the door for him he told me how beautiful I looked. I felt nervous and told him that it was the Retin-A cream I was using. He said 'Gee whiz, you must give me some of that cream!'"

To your loved ones, you are always young. The facelift is so natural that everyone adjusts to your looking younger. With the passage of time, your brain will also discard the aged image in favor of the younger one. That is the mark of good artistic surgery.

BRAVADO IN BRAZIL

CARLOS OSCAR UEBEL, M.D.
PORTO ALEGRE, BRAZIL

Be bloody, bold, and resolute.
–William Shakespeare

Our plastic surgery clinic in Porto Alegre, Brazil, is fanatical in its pursuit of two goals: the rigid observance of its aseptic procedures and care of the patient. Because these goals are consistently met, our highly competent surgeons and nurses are able to deploy their skills in achieving extremely high success rates in all our procedures.

One of the elements in this practice is to exclude all non-professionals from the operating room – even patients' friends and relatives. This might seem to be a somewhat harsh and unyielding policy, but our experience has been that it pays off in terms of absence of pathogens circulating in pre-operational environment, and therefore of minimizing postoperative infection risks. Of course, doctors and nurses, including those who might be related to (or friends of) patients are admitted.

We are even more strict in applying this rule to the operation itself. Apart from the asepsis aspect, the last thing the surgical team would want is any disturbance to the practiced regularity of a procedure.

These regulations worked well for us over a period of years, until one day a woman came in to have breast implants. Problem was, her husband showed up and asked for permission to take video shots of the surgery; he wanted to show his wife and family how the procedure was done. His timing could not have been worse. The lady was already in the OR, the anesthesiologist beginning the epidural block.

I planted myself in front of the husband.

"Sir, I'm afraid that your request cannot be granted. It is simply impossible to go against the precedent that has been in force for so many years. First, it would upset the OR routine. Second, you could be the source of contamination and therefore of sepsis. Third – and most important of all – you might start feeling ill or giddy, even faint. You've never been present at a surgical operation, and the fact that the subject is your own wife makes it all the more difficult to observe dispassionately."

His attitude became combative.

"Doctor, I've served as a captain in the Brazilian army. I've survived jungle rescue missions. I've fought alligators, stabbed large predatory cats, and killed immense jiboia snakes. It's fair to say that I'm a brave man, doctor, and under extreme conditions I've had my share of visualizing and feeling the blood running from wounds in my own body."

His voice had risen to a scream, and his last words were in a loud begging tone.

"Please, please let me in."

We were faced with a difficult situation. The man seemed capable of causing a disruption outside the OR and certainly of engaging our attention, which should have been focused on the patient. By now, the anesthesiologist had called us to say that he was ready for us to begin the operation, which would take about an hour. With some misgivings, I chose the lesser of two evils and decided to let him in to see the procedure, make his brief "documentary," and then quietly leave.

After a short discussion with the nursing director, we got the husband quickly scrubbed up and into surgical clothing and moved him into a corner of the room where he could begin running his camera.

At first, everything went according to the well-rehearsed routine. We began the surgery, incising and cauterizing. The team worked together like a machine in the near-silent, aseptic environment of the operating room. It had all the signs of being a completely normal procedure.

Then it happened. There was a deafening crash from the corner, and we all turned away from the patient to see our valorous army captain lying on the floor, with a four-inch laceration his scalp gushing an unhindered flow of blood. Beside him lay the ruined video camera.

He was cold. Quickly one of the doctors knelt beside him and applied stimuli, to which he did not react. Without warning, the husband had become the priority patient. The wife was still fully anesthetized, so we left her under the care of the senior theater nurse while we handled the new emergency.

We carried him awkwardly into the adjacent recovery room and began life-saving maneuvers. We cleared the obstructions to his breathing passages, inserted an endotracheal tube through which we could administer oxygen, injected saline solution, compressed the wound to staunch the blood flow, and sutured the yawning gash.

It took two hours before our second patient began to regain consciousness, when one of our specialists decided that we could safely withdraw the endotracheal tube. We were all more than relieved when the husband began to babble enough words that we could understand. He was asking what had happened.

During this time, out primary patient had awakened from the diminishing effects of the anesthetic. She was confused and upset because she could hear the uproar in the recovery room. Like her husband, she too was anxiously questioning what was going on.

Eventually, the damaged captain was stable enough to be left under the observation of a nurse, and we returned to the OR. The anesthesiologist infused more anesthetic through the peridural catheter, reinforced by a sedative, so we were able to continue our surgery in the appropriate calm environment.

Late in the afternoon, husband and wife were both in the recovery room. She was overjoyed at the success of her mammary prosthesis. He, on the contrary, lay with an enormous helmet to cover his damaged scalp, the very picture of embarrassment and contrition.

From the time of this tragicomedy on, we never again allowed such intrusion into the sanctity of our operating room, Amazon jungle adventurers included.

Bravado may be all very well in the right circumstances, but not in the surroundings of a plastic surgery operation.

THOROUGH EXAM

JAMES BAKER, M.D.   WINTER PARK, FL

Truth is beautiful, without doubt;
and so are lies.
–Emerson

In the early '70s, when I was one of the first plastic surgeons in Florida doing office surgery, patients found out they could have a breast enlargement done without the stigma of going to a hospital and, through word of mouth, the interest spread rapidly. As a result, I was doing a vast number of breast augmentations in the office as an outpatient procedure.

I had a young nurse when I first went into practice who came from a very religious family and had married a Lutheran minister. She was quite a "prim and proper" young lady.

As was our custom, we would bring the post-op augmentation patients in one after the other for their check-ups. We had four examining rooms down a corridor, and each room was a mirror image of the other. I would walk in the examining room and sitting on the edge of the examing table would be a young lady with a paper gown top which, in the essence of time, I would remove, grab the breasts and squeeze them to see if there was any firmness developing. I was most interested in the problem of capsule or contracture and was trying to come up with reasons for why it occurred. I would grasp the breasts and, if they were soft, I would say, "They feel great," and then go to the next room, and so on. I would dictate the charts after the four patients in the consecutive rooms had left.

I reached the fourth examining room, and there was a very attractive young lady sitting on the edge of the table, just as there had been in the previous three rooms. I pulled the paper gown off, grabbed her breasts, and said, "Gee, these feel great." I looked at my nurse, who had a dumbfounded, fearful expression on her face, and looked back at the patient, who looked rather confused. My nurse then quickly interjected that this was a new patient and she was here for moles on her back. I immediately looked her in the eyes and said, "Well, that's fine. The breasts have no lumps in them." I then went to examine her back and advised her that none of the lesions appeared malignant, but that we could remove them for cosmetic reasons if she desired. She looked at me and said that she was very impressed since I was the only doctor she'd ever been to who took the time to examine her breasts for lumps. Obviously, at 23 years of age there would have been no need for such an exam.

The patient left feeling like she had had a very thorough doctor examining her, and I felt very relieved that my nurse had alerted me to the situation as quickly as she did.

LOOK BEFORE YOU LEAP

JAMES W. MAY, JR., M.D.   BOSTON, MA

A wise man sees as much as he ought,
not as much as he can.
–Montaigne

In my plastic surgery clinic at the Massachusetts General Hospital, it is my usual practice to have the patient's record posted in a small bracket on the examination room door. This gives me an opportunity to review the chart briefly before going into the room.

One particularly busy day, I picked the chart from its bracket, but I did not take the time to review it before walking into the exam room. I saw a man in his mid-twenties sitting in the patient chair and immediately noticed a very prominent characteristic: his right ear, which protruded ninety degrees from the mastoid region. His left ear was essentially normal in external configuration.

I greeted the waiting patient. Then while making small talk with him on superficial topics, I gave intense thought to the fascinating challenge of subtly refining the position of his right ear so as to match the appearance of the normal left ear. It must have been obvious to him from the intensity of my observation of his errant ear that it was the focus of my examination.

He broke into our conversation. "Doctor, are you thinking that this appointment is about correction of my right ear?"

"Why, I . . . er . . ." I stopped short, realizing that I had neither asked him why he had come to see me, nor had I even looked at his record. I now looked at the chart and saw that his appointment was to see me for the removal of a small mole on his upper chest. He was not the least interested in my opinions, let alone the correction of his right ear.

Look – and listen – before you leap!

THE MISSING NIPPLE

LUIS VASCONEZ, M.D.   BIRMINGHAM, AL

Trivials make perfection, but perfection is not trivial.
—Michelangelo

We were doing a large breast reduction on a lady, using an inferior pedicle – a piece of tissue to support the nipple. As we proceeded with the operation, specimens of unwanted tissue which had been removed were passed to the circulating nurse for disposal.

We were taken by surprise when, having temporarily closed the left breast with staples, we were unable to locate the nipple. Where could it be?

"Oh, my God, the nipple must be here," exclaimed the nurse, pointing at the unwanted tissue. "It must have been passed to me as not needed!"

Chills ran simultaneously down all our spines, and our state of mind became near-catatonic.

I said to the nurse, "Let's find it. Perhaps we can use it as a free-graft."

She unfolded the specimens. No nipple.

There was nothing to do but re-open the left breast and investigate. Mercifully, we found that the nipple had been folded with the long inferior pedicle.

The team's relief was palpable!

JUMPING TO CONCLUSIONS

NARENDRA PANDYA, M.D.
BOMBAY, INDIA

Errare humanum est.
Anonymous

Alexander Pope assures us that while to err is human, to forgive is divine. In many walks of life, the principle of forgiveness for mistakes made is admirable and, in many cases, practicable. The field of medicine, however, is one in which errors are least likely to be condoned. The stakes are too high.

After twenty-five years experience in the field of plastic surgery, I believed that I had fine-tuned my practice to a point where I had reduced to a minimum my human propensity to err in professional matters. How wrong I was.

I had known for some years a married lady who moved in the upper echelons of Bombay society. She was a poised and elegant woman of thirty or so, active and successful in several charitable organizations. She was politically active, too, and had made a bid for office in the state assembly. Invariably well dressed, her clothes always emphasized her lovely figure. All around, an attractive and accomplished woman, who would have deserved the accolade of "beautiful" except for one thing.

Her nose.

This one feature was so extraordinarily ugly that it seemed to dominate her whole appearance. It was large, it was ill-

15

shaped, it was a mess. On the many occasions that I had the opportunity to meet and converse with her socially, the professional compartment of my mind would go into action, working on the ways and means that plastic surgery could help her escape from this predicament. Fuel would be added to this fire on these occasions, because she would invariably break off from the subject of conversation to say: "Dr. Pandya, I must come and see you – I'm so concerned about a personal problem that I'm sure you could help me with."

But for a long time she did not follow up her comment with a visit to my office, and the whole matter seemed to fade from her mind until, inevitably, the next time we met it would come up again. As I saw her quite frequently, I found myself becoming almost obsessed with the awfulness of this lady's nose, and I couldn't help wondering if she would ever reach a decision to ask for my help.

One evening she and I found ourselves together at a gathering of friends. I was disturbed at her appearance: Her usual poise seemed to be fraying at the edges, she was nervous, upset almost. She made a beeline for me, and got straight to the point. Her voice was agitated.

"Doctor, I have to see you. I mustn't put off this problem any longer. It just won't wait. Will you see me tomorrow?"

Her look was imploring.

"Of course. I have a fairly full program tomorrow, but I'll be free by late afternoon. Why don't you just call the young lady in my office early in the morning, and we'll set up the consultation right away."

And so we did. At five the following evening, she sat opposite me at my desk. Well presented as ever, she seemed to have regained her poise – the result, it seemed to me, of having made up her mind to have something done about that dreadful nose. She came straight to the point.

"I've been hesitating for a long time – years, in fact – to come see you about this problem that is troubling me so much. But now I'm determined to go ahead and ask for your professional help."

Instead of replying, I just nodded, hoping to convey my agreement with her decision and to indicate my full support. As she went on, I was picturing in my mind's eye what the end result would be after I'd taken off the huge hump, reduced the over-large tip, and brought the nostrils into proportion.

"You see, doctor, the reason I've been putting this consultation off for so long is that my husband thinks I'm stupid to worry about such a thing. Those of my friends I've confided in feel the same way. And now . . . now, I just hope that you don't think me stupid as well, to be so concerned about what might seem to you an unimportant physical problem. You don't, do you, doctor?"

She looked anxiously at me.

I was about to reply with words of reassurance that I could tame that unfortunate nose, that one great imperfection in her otherwise perfect appearance. But before the words came out, she dropped a bomb.

"You see, doctor, my breasts are so small that I find them an embarrassment. Every time I try on new clothes, every time I go out, every time I'm with . . . with my husband . . .," she swallowed, hesitated, and then went on. " . . . I feel so much less than a complete woman."

I was stopped in my tracks. To think that after all my years of practice I was capable of making such a fundamental error of judgment! My patient's concern was totally different from what I wrongly assumed. I was confused, but at the same time, relieved that I had not made the even worse mistake of putting my thoughts into words. I turned a mental somersault and hoped that she would not sense any hint of my miscalculation when I spoke.

"Far from being stupid, I think that you are very wise to come to a decision that can so relieve your state of mind. It is very common for a young woman like you who has small breasts to be concerned – you are not alone in your worries.

"And of course I can help. The procedure we will consider is known as augmentation mammoplasty. It is routine surgery, with the highest possible chance of excellent results. Now, let me do an initial examination."

Just two weeks later, I performed the operation. Everything went well, and the outcome was a complete success.

I have met this lady several times since. She never tires of telling me how happy she and her husband are, how completely her life has changed for the better, how much more confident and comfortable she feels with her body.
She is, in short, a contented woman.

The nose – that unsightly appendage to an otherwise lovely face – the nose is still there, for all to see. The fuller breasts, though, are known only to herself, her husband, and me.

As for me, I continue to chastise myself for that gross error, the error of miscalculating a person's needs. Even after long practice in the field of plastic surgery, *errare humanum est.* It was just good fortune for me that I never put that miscalculation into words. If I had, divine forgiveness would certainly have been required.

TRADING UP

PETER BELA FODOR, M.D.
LOS ANGELES, CA

Two elements are needed to form a truth,
a fact and an abstraction.
–Gourmont

A highpowered executive in his late 50s came in for facial restorative surgery. His primary aim was to look as young as possible. It was decided that a facelift, nose job, upper and lower lids, and otoplasty (the pinning back of the ears) would be appropriate.

Three months after surgery, the patient took his wife to a Broadway show. During intermission, a friend walked past them several times without saying hello. It was obvious from her body language that she was trying to avoid them. The patient returned to his seat while his wife went to the ladies room.

As the wife was returning to her seat, she bumped into the friend. After some awkward small talk, the friend commented that she hadn't realized that she and her husband were no longer together. She found it remarkable that her current escort looked so much like her husband – only younger – and proceeded to state that she was proud of the fact that nowadays women as well as men can trade up for a younger partner.

THE EYE OF THE STORM

BARRY ZIDE, M.D.   NEW YORK, NY

No man is exempt from silly things;
the mischief is to say them deliberately.
–Montaigne

When she called me from her Long Island home, the woman sounded more than concerned; distressed is a better word. She told me that her husband had been in an automobile accident some three months earlier, suffering what sounded like a severe eye injury. She asked for an urgent evaluation of the scar around the orbital region which was causing him a lot of misery. She sounded so disturbed that I juggled some of my calendar times, and they arrived in my office later that afternoon.

I had expected to see a pretty massive injury, "an orbital scar from an automobile accident." Actually, it was nothing more than a one-centimeter, well-healed laceration of the eyebrow. I was perplexed. Why the urgency, what was the problem?

The wife spoke. "Do you think that this scar should keep us from having sexual intercourse?"

"No, of course not," I replied

"Well, it has for the last three months." She turned to her husband, and continued, "you son-of-a-bitch, you're having an affair," and raised her hand to slap him. As quickly as it takes to read these words, I found myself in the middle of a domestic dispute.

21

I stood up. "Hey, guys – you have to figure this out some-place else, not in my office," and escorted them both to the door.

The wife had used me not as a medical adviser, but as a proving ground to expose her husband's philandering. Wild!

THE HUMAN TORCH

ROBERT N. COOPER, M.D.   STUART, FL

Burnt child fire dreadeth.
–John Heywood

My surgery center in Florida is a concrete-and-steel struc-
ture of 20,000 square feet overlooking to the north a sweep-
ing panorama over Stuart's St. Lucie River. It is of massive
construction, and is essentially hurricane-proof, bullet-proof,
and, most importantly, fireproof.

This was not always the case. My previous facility, just a
couple of blocks east of the current one, was a much older
building, concrete on the lower floor but wooden on the
upper. It lacked a sprinkler system and thus could not qualify for the practice of surgery. Then in May 1994 an event
took place which taught me a lesson in fire hazard that I've
never forgotten.

Raymond and his wife, Denise, came to me in Florida for
simultaneous eyelid and facelift surgery, and checked into
the upper annex of the older building. Their procedures were
uneventful and, subsequently, they were taken to their two-
bedroom apartment. Both made good, rapid recoveries.
Raymond, although a heavy smoker, had stopped two weeks
earlier, much to the benefit of his healing process.

I made a housecall on them that first evening and found
everything to be totally satisfactory. I drove home in a
relaxed frame of mind, with no thought of trouble ahead.

3:25 a.m. is not the best time to be awakened from a deep

sleep with an emergency call.   "Dr. Cooper, you have a patient on fire in the annex!"

The cobwebs of sleep immediately cleared.   "Just repeat that, would you?"

"Your patient is on fire!"

I dressed as I ran to my car. I gunned the engine, skidded out of the driveway, and reached close to 100 mph during the five-mile ride. I was aware of fire engines screaming their off-key sirens, and my mind filled with terrible visions of my patients' charred bodies being pulled out of the burning annex.

I slid the car to a jolting stop in front of the building and was just slightly relieved to see that it looked still intact. I raced ahead of the young firemen who had arrived at the same moment, opened the front door, and walked into a wall of choking smoke. I clawed through the acrid fog, found the door to Raymond's room wide open, and charged in.

Raymond, only minimally agitated, was standing in the middle of the room, visible through the now slowly clearing smoke. His head dressing was singed and lay on the smoldering carpet. He was talking to one of the private duty nurses. It was a surreal, nightmarish scene.

It transpired that an hour earlier Raymond had found that he could not sleep without the benefit of a cigarette. He stepped into the living room, taking with him a pack of coffin nails and his lighter.

My practice in those days was to dress the faces of the patients with cotton held in place by a fishnet dressing, open at mid-face to expose eyes, nose, and mouth. When Raymond lit up, he achieved a NASA-like ignition and liftoff of this highly flammable material, effectively catching fire to his face.

He tore off the burning dressing in time to keep his personal damage to a superficial second degree burn on the cheeks. But the burning carpet created the smoke, which raised the alarm. He had the presence of mind to stamp out the carpet fire with his leather slippers.

When I burst in, he was at once terrified and embarrassed, and offered immediate penance in the form of paying for a new carpet.

On my part, my experience of fire risk moved immediately from the theoretical to the severely practical. My visions of burned patients did not turn out to be true, but since then my precautions have always been heavily weighted on the side of fire prevention.

BUREAUCRACY

S.E. THORVALDSSON, M.D.
REYKJAVIK, ICELAND

Nothing is there more friendly
to a man, than a friend in need.
–Titus Maccius Plautus

Iceland may seem a remote and strange land to most of the world, but in fact its society much resembles that of any western nation. When I came to the United States to pursue my medical studies, I found the same mix of the pleasant and unpleasant, the good and the bad, the easy and the difficult, as any visitor would find in my native country.

I was well prepared to appreciate an experience which had little to do with plastic surgery per se, but everything to do with helpfulness, friendship, and forbearance. It happened to me when I was about to start my plastic surgery residency in Ann Arbor, Michigan.

Dr. Damon was in charge of the program. He and his wife, Thelma, were the key people in a minor drama that played out for me in my first week in Ann Arbor. I first met them at a barbecue party which was held by the graduating residents for the incoming group, to help them make the acquaintance of the more senior doctors and of the staff. I met Dr. Damon and his wife, and we talked about generalities until I mentioned that I had not yet had the time or opportunity to buy a car.

Dr. Damon immediately said, "Sigi, I have two cars. Why

26

don't you borrow one of them? Thelma, I'm sure, won't mind driving me to work, will you, dear?"

His wife smiled her agreement. I felt hesitant about accepting this friendly gesture. But after only the briefest of moments to consider (I really needed that car!), I replied, "Doctor Damon, that's very good of you. If it's really no trouble to you, I'll take advantage of your kind offer. I hope it will be for only a short time, until I have a car of my own."

Three days later I had finished my shopping around and decided on the car I wanted to buy. I didn't know it then, but that was just the beginning of my struggle with all the regulations and accompanying paperwork. I needed to have a driver's license, which I hadn't yet qualified for, but to take the test I had to own a car in which to be tested.

I couldn't buy the car unless I had insurance; so, driving Dr. Damon's big blue station wagon very carefully, I made my way to the AAA office to persuade them to let me have insurance on a car that I hadn't yet bought.

Leaving the borrowed station wagon parked outside the building, I went in and was soon engaged in trying to explain this increasingly complex situation to the young gentleman in charge of business. After fifteen minutes of weaving our way through the bureaucratic fog, we were interrupted by a young lady who came running breathlessly into the office.

"Does anyone here have a big blue station wagon parked out front?" Her voice was anxious, agitated.

I looked up. "Yes, I do."

"Well, I just ran into it. It's a wreck."

I froze. I visualized with appalling clarity what would now unfold. Before even starting my residency, the car that I had borrowed from the program director had been wrecked. I was sure that there would be no need for me to show up for the first day of work, as that would also be the last one as far as I was concerned. I envisioned calling IcelandAir to book the next available seat on a flight home.

When I had regained enough composure to move, the first thing, of course, was to go out and look at the car. It had suffered a lot of body damage, but was probably drivable. Next action was to exchange insurance and other information with the girl who caused the collision. Finally, I had to call Dr. Damon and to give him the bad news.

"May I use your telephone?" I asked the AAA agent.

"Please – go right ahead."

When the call went through, the doctor wasn't in the office. His secretary asked me if the message was important, and I felt that I could safely say that it was.

"You can leave a message on his answering machine," said the secretary.

I had the unenviable task of recording the story of how his new resident had already wrecked his car. I found that very difficult, as I would have much preferred to speak to him directly and get it over with.

It turned out that the car was capable of being driven safely. The damage, although extensive, was mainly cosmetic –

and would obviously be costly to fix. I took it back to the clinic the next day, went into his office, and started again explaining what had happened.

I had hardly begun when he interrupted.

"Look, Sigi, there's nothing you could have done about it. It was just sitting there."

And that was the end of the matter.

This was how I came quickly to learn of Dr. Damon's well-deserved reputation as a father-figure to all the residents. His kindness on this embarrassing occasion underscored the esteem in which he was held by his trainees.

What I feared would be the terminating disaster of my residency even before it began, set the tone for the next two years. Dr. Damon's tolerance and leadership were the hallmark of that course, and he was always respected, never feared, by the residents. His friendly humanity is my most precious memory of the entire training period.

THE STALKER

WALDEMAR F. HERRMANN, M.D.
MINEOLA, NY

The ardor chills us which we do not share.
—Patmore

I had never met seventy-something Mary until she came into my office asking for liposuction. She wanted to have a lump on thigh and buttocks removed. The background to the case was that she had been hit by a car and developed a hematoma, which had developed over several years into a lipomatous lump, a large benign tumor of fat cells.

During the recitation of her problem she grew very excited, and said that she had heard a lot about me. So agitated did she become, in fact, that her explanation degenerated into what could only be described as ranting and raving. She was what is popularly termed a motor-mouth. She talked so fast and so much that I could hardly get a word in to ask the necessary questions. The consultation became virtually a one-way street, and she became increasingly anxious to emphasize the reality of her complaint. When her flow of words seemed inadequate, she finally said: "Here, I will show you."

Then, with no further ado, she began to take her clothes off, with nothing between the two of us and the outside world but the unlocked office door. It began as an embarrassing situation and turned into a sickening one. Quite clearly, her underwear had not been washed for a month, and her last bath or shower must have been long before that. Her belly-button was a black spot; she had dirty streaks in her groin and on her belly. Sure enough, she had lumps on the lateral thigh and the lower buttocks, but at the time I could focus only on her unclean state.

I had to bring some order into a deteriorating situation. I went to my desk, riffled through a number of random papers, then said to her, "I can't find the necessary document to record all your complaints – I'll have to get it from outside. Stay here while I find one"

As with many surgeons, it is my practice to keep printed sheets with outline drawings of a body and various body parts, which make it easier to document and record all my findings. I found the one I was looking for and then turned to my nurse, asking her to go into my office and rescue me from the nutty, near-naked female. The nurse went in and threw a towel around my difficult patient. Then she took her into a treatment room, where we charted all of her wounds and documented them on the relevant sheet.

Mary had another problem. After the accident, she had received financial compensation for the injuries she'd received. This money, however, she blew on other things than her physical well-being, and ended up broke. Hence she was on Medicaid; but Medicaid would not pay for a procedure which was considered to be cosmetic.

I made a few phone calls and succeeded in convincing the medical provider that this was not a cosmetic procedure but a posttraumatic one which would relieve her discomfort and, sometimes, pain. So the financial way was made clear for surgery to be made feasible.

We booked her for surgery, which in due course was carried out uneventfully. After recovery, Mary seemed happy about the way everything had gone.

But that's not quite the end of the story.

Some time after the Mary episode, I suffered a bout of illness and a heart attack. These misfortunes persuaded me to quit practice and, instead, to take over as medical director of a surgical center that we owned.

Unbelievable as it may sound, Mary tracked me down, and came to my new office to do the same thing she did before.

As she explained it, she had undergone some gynecological surgery through what is known as a Pfannenstiel incision – along the line of the lower part of a bikini costume – and was unhappy with the scar. She had been to a plastic surgeon to improve the scar. The surgeon told her that the scar amelioration alone would not do the trick and that a belly-lift would be needed to make the result much better.

That, of course, meant more money; her financial position had not improved, and she couldn't pay for the belly-lift. So the plastic surgeon had gone ahead and improved the scar, omitting the belly-lift procedure.

The result: a very nice scar in an overhanging lap of fatty tissue and skin.

Having found me, Mary went into her previous routine. Right in my office, door unlocked, she pulled her pants down to show me the result. Against her unstoppable flow of words, I finally convinced her that she just had to have a belly-lift done, and that was that.

"Yeah," she said, "but he wanted so much money, and I didn't want to pay for it, so he just did the scar without the belly-lift."

Her clothing was in the same disarray as the first time, and there was no improvement at all in the area or personal hygiene. And as for that belly-button . . .!

In a plastic surgery environment, one meets all sorts and conditions of people, but Mary was the most unforgettable of my patients. She tried, on several more occasions to track me down in my office; but, I had instructed the front desk that whenever she showed up I was unavailable, in a meeting.

She finally got the message. She was unwanted.

THE PURITY Of YOUTH

ROBERT N. COOPER, M.D.   STUART, FL

How awful to reflect that what people say of us is true.
–L. P. Smith

About twelve years ago, I had occasion to meet in consultation a very attractive 60-year-old female. She was one of those women gifted with a marvelous set of genes. At the time of her consultation, she looked like she was in her early 40s. Unfortunately, some women, given such a gift, are highly critical of themselves.

They have always seen themselves as quite attractive, and I've found over the years that their tolerance of imperfection is quite small. Therefore, their threshold for intervention is rather low. They have always had this gift of good looks and, like a measure of security tucked away in a back pocket, they could always rely upon it. This particular lady was given a very substantial gift, and yet I felt that her expectations and request for facial rejuvenation were reasonable.

Postoperatively, she enjoyed a fabulous result. No one could have accurately judged her age to be 60. She looked like she was in her late 30s, maybe 40 years of age. The great preponderance of that was probably genetic and not from virtuoso surgical skill.

She did, however, relate a story that has become one of the favorites generated from my practice. She told me that she had been in an exclusive boutique shop when she asked her four-year-old grandson to come to her, so she could show him something. At that moment, that shopkeeper looked at her quizzically. Apparently, my patient had said to the young boy, "Come here, Jimmy, Grandma wants to show you something."

The shopkeeper apparently could not believe that she was the grandmother of this young boy. She deftly and somewhat delicately approached my patient and suggested that the young boy could not possibly be my patient's grandson.

Apparently, a polite exchange went back and forth between the two ladies, one woman asserting, "He certainly is my grandson," and the other lady contending, "How could a woman as young as you have a grandson?" The flattering banter of the shopkeeper could possibly have had an ulterior motive, but, taking it at face value, the back-and-forth exchange proceeded until my patient squared up in front of the shopkeeper and politely declared, "This is my grandson. Thank you for your flattering remarks, but my son is 40 years old."

Later that evening, at a dinner table hosting the entire longitudinal family of three generations, my patient was relating this story. Her grown children were laughing and enjoying the dilemma of their mother declaring that she was older than she appeared, and that it was quite fitting that this young child be her grandson. The teasing and laughter had only gone on for a short time before the young grandson sensed there was something wrong. He abruptly got up from the table and walked around to where his grandmother was seated. He picked up his little hand and petted her hand, looking her in the face quite seriously. Looking down at him, she saw that he was troubled and, before she could say anything, he attempted to comfort her by saying. "It's okay,

Grandma, you still look old to me."

The purity and innocence of youth had led the young boy to reassure his Grandma that she still looked old. Obviously, he thought there was something quite wrong with looking too young.

It remains one of the favorite stories of my practice.

TOP SECRET

STEPHEN HOEFFLIN, M.D.
SANTA MONICA, CA

The young man knows the rules,
but the old man knows the exceptions.
−Oliver Wendell Holmes

As plastic surgeons, we all understand and respect the confidentiality desired by our patients − none more so than people such as VIPs, celebrities, and politicians to whom it is of the first importance.

One of my patients, however, a prominent European woman, carried this need for privacy to an altogether higher level. She wanted a face-lift, but specified that all written and telephone communication betwen herself and my California office was to be conducted with the utmost secrecy. The reason? Simple: Her husband, equally prominent in Europe, did not approve of plastic surgery, and so she wanted the procedure carried through entirely without his knowledge.

She made arrangements to stay at a Beverly Hills hotel under an assumed name, accompanied by one of her girlfriends. She and her husband were accustomed to being protected by bodyguards, but she refused any such protection. She went so far as to request that consultations in my office should be conducted at night so as to minimize any risk of being spotted in daylight hours. The whole thing assumed the likeness of a CIA operation rather than a routine surgical procedure.

How did she explain her absence to her husband? She told him that she was going on a several-week shopping spree in Beverly Hills with her lady friend, and that he might well not hear from her for a period of time because she was going to be "too busy." Nothing could have been better calculated to arouse his suspicions.

Her cover was not blown. Neither the hotel nor anyone in my office had any idea who she was. I went ahead with the face-lift procedure, which went well. I saw her during her brief stay in a postoperative recovery center and then in her hotel suite.

Although everything had run smoothly to that point, I was still concerned that her need for privacy had precluded any information going to her husband. She convinced me that her insistence on being so secretive was simply to avoid any unpleasantness with him, and she assured me that this was frequently the way of handling things in her own country.

International media coverage, availability of information on the Internet, and frank acknowledgments by European people of high visibility that they had undergone cosmetic surgery have ensured that acceptance of cosmetic surgery has gained ground in Europe over the years. However, there are still certain countries where it is frowned upon, and my patient came from one of them. So I kept my concerns to myself and charged myself and my staff to protect her confidentiality to the greatest extent possible.

On the patient's fifth postoperative day, I made an evening visit to the Beverly Hills hotel. As I got out of the elevator, I noticed that a large man was following me. My guess was that he was a member of hotel security; but I had second thoughts when it seemed that he was taking a photograph from the end of the hallway as I entered the lady's room. I removed a few sutures, gave her some words of reassurance and instructions, and left her suite.

The man was gone.

As I drove away, I had a strange feeling that a car followed me from the hotel for some distance, but I dismissed the thought as being fanciful.

Then two evenings later, I returned to the hotel to check on my patient once more. This time there were two men in the corridor leading to her room – the original bruiser and a new one. I mentioned this to the lady, her girlfriend (who was still staying with her) followed up by saying that there appeared to be a large number of security guards around the hotel. This was not unusual in Beverly Hills, although the two individuals in the corridor did not fit the pattern.

The layout of the suite consisted of a living area and two separate bedrooms. I was removing a few more sutures, with the friend watching me, when the door opened and the two men burst in. Shock and disbelief registered on all our faces, followed by recognition by my patient that the larger gentleman was her husband's head of security. It was quickly obvious that he realized that he was looking at a postoperative scenario, and she was not doing what her husband had suspected: having an affair with a younger man in a Beverly Hills hotel.

We all sat down and put the whole story together, with confidentiality abandoned. The husband's suspicions had been so thoroughly aroused that he had managed to monitor the telephone calls and faxes between my patient and my office, which made him more certain that some shady business was going on. He sent his head of security to keep tabs on her; when he observed a man entering her room in the evenings, he called the husband and was ordered to enter the room. It was evident, although never confirmed, that one of the hotel employees was paid off to obtain a pass-key.

The occasions when I entered the patient's room late at night solidified his worst suspicions, and he gave the order to enter the room on the assumption that she was having a secret affair. He had no idea that she was having a secret facelift.

The story has a happy ending. The husband flew in to California and came to the hotel. My patient, her girlfriend, the husband, and I had a conversation which was, to put it mildly, strained in the early stages. Everything was eventually sorted out, the husband accepted the situation with good grace, and the four of us ended up as friends.

I continue to guard my patients' confidentiality with due diligence. Never again, though, will I allow it to reach these levels of international intrigue.They are too liable to backfire on the patient – and on me.

BOARD CERTIFYING EXAMINATION

TIMOTHY MILLER, M.D.
LOS ANGELES, CA

A fool is his own informer.
—Yiddish Proverb

The Board examination is a common experience of plastic surgeons. Its two phases – the written and the oral - are equally demanding, both emotionally and intellectually. Where they differ is in the level of stress, where the oral produces anxiety on an order of magnitude greater than the written.

My examination was held in New York City's splendid Waldorf Astoria, although my financial standing required that I stay with the three other candidates in a much less impressive hotel. The four of us occupied two adjoining rooms with an interconnecting door.

When I arrived, I had come to the firm conclusion that there would be no point in final, last-minute study before the exam. I had been hitting the books for many months, and would use these last few hours to relax and to go clear-headed into the oral inquisition. My plan was to take a run in the park, enjoy a quiet dinner, have a good night's sleep.

Those ideas went out the window soon after there was a knock on the door to the connected room.

I opened the door, and there stood one of my fellow examinees, his eyes locked on the thick wad of notes tightly grasped in his hand.

"When collagen cross-links, does it involve an aldehyde bond?" he said, without raising his stare at the pages.

My silence made him look up at my face. "You all right?" he asked, concerned.

"Yeah, sure. I – ah – think – yes, aldehyde bonds are involved . . . ."

"Vanderwahl electrical stuff keeps going through my head," he continued. He looked down again at the notebook, at least five inches thick. "They covered it in the review course."

As clearly as the life's events of a drowning man are supposed to run through his mind, I had a vision of my decision not to take the review course. My stomach felt as though I were in an elevator that had suddenly dropped four floors.

But it got worse. I had not brought any notes, just a copy of Grabb and Smith which, I might add, had absolutely nothing about collagen's role in wound healing.

My voice became a whisper. "You know, to be honest . . .I just don't remember."

"That could be painful for you." This from a man I considered to be my friend!

"You take the exam at ten in the morning, right?" I had given him this information earlier. "What if Earl Peacock is your examiner?"

My drowning man syndrome became more acute, probably helped by the sudden and disproportionate weight distribution caused by the slippage of my abdominal contents to somewhere deep in the rectus femoris muscles.

"Well," I muttered, "I won't have much say in that." My next door neighbor turned around and retreated into his room, leaving me to close the door and fall supine on my bed. My mind was capable of nothing more than counting the individual white beads of the ceiling tiles. Sort of a poor man's mantra.

The count completed, I grabbed the textbook, then thumbed through its pages. As an aid to increasing my pre-exam knowledge, it didn't mean a lot, but at least I succeeded in calming myself for a few minutes until the next knock on the door, this time the one leading into the corridor.

It was my roommate, and within a few minutes our conversation predictably moved to the upcoming examination.

"Glad I took that course" he said proudly. He pulled from his suitcase a notebook similar to the one I'd seen next door, again quite remarkably thick. He had gone a step further, having inserted colored tabs to help him quickly identify different topics.

We went on talking for a few minutes, but in the end

I couldn't resist the temptation to ask him about the subject that had floored me. I made my voice sound as casual as I could, and asked "Anything in there about collagen cross-linkage?"

The way his fingers flew over the tabs reminded me of a blackjack dealer in Vegas. Within seconds, the notebook was open at the precise page he was looking for. Without a word, he turned the book toward me. There was a colored diagram of the collagen molecule which effortlessly described cross-linkage, the chemical pathways by which it occurred, and how it could be blocked.

The connecting door opened again – no knock, this time. Greetings all round, but almost immediately it was three of them, the ones who had taken the course, the ones I'd thought of as friends, and one of me, the uninformed outsider. They talked among themselves of how to sit in the exam room and how best to phrase their answers. They discussed surgical procedures I'd never heard of, a conversation so foreign to me that they might as well have been speaking Russian.

To his great credit, my roommate realized there was a problem.

"Would you like to review my notes on collagen?" My plans for a relaxing dinner disappeared, but his words earned my eternal gratitude. By midnight, I had learned more in five hours than I seemed to have read in the previous several months. All I had to do now was to remember this material.

A run! That would do it.

"Could you direct me to Central Park?" This to the doorman, who was sitting by the locked front door.

"What did you have in mind?" he asked as only a New Yorker could, eying my shoes, sweat pants, and shirt. "Do you want to run through it or around it?"

"Either" I replied casually. "What would be the difference?"

"If a young man wanted to commit suicide but didn't care t

too much how the end came, you know, the actual method of dying, you could run through the Park at this hour. Otherwise, I would suggest running around it, and do it as quickly as you can."

So much for the idea of a stress-releasing run.

My sleep that night was fitful, but the designated time found me outside the exam room taking deep, relaxing breaths. I had managed to bring myself to a strong six on a calmness scale of one to ten – at least, until the previous candidate came out.

He was a USA Army major, wearing dark green dress uniform. But neither the dark shade of his clothing nor the dim light of the hallway could conceal the fact that the sweat had made its way right through the back and front of his jacket. His face was ashen. He walked past me with his face frozen in a look of horror.

On rubbery legs, I entered the room and immediately recognized one of my two examiners. He and I had talked together two weeks before, at the University of Arizona. His reputation was that of being one of the most intelligent plastic surgery educators and surgeons. He was quick, he was bright, and – I had to admit to myself – he was inspiring.

His name was Earl Peacock.

He greeted me warmly, and introduced his co-examiner, whose name I cannot recall to this day.

"Well, let's get down to it, shall we?" Dr. Peacock's voice was friendly and informal. I nodded, steeling myself for a cross-linkage question for which I had every conceivable answer, provided only that I could remember my roommate's notes.

It was not to be. "Dr. Miller, what is the most common cause of unilateral nasal drainage in a five-year old child?"

The answer was not in Grabb and Smith, nor was it in the notes that my roommate had so generously lent me. I could sense that the examination that would determine much of my future life was already heading downhill, and the slope was steep.

I offered tumors, a deviated septum, even a common cold. In a word, I was floundering badly. Dr. Peacock told me the answer he wanted to hear.

"A green pea he took from his brother's plate at lunch."

The metaphor of slippery slope was replaced by that of quicksand. I was already in it up to mid-thigh.

"Well, let's move on." The examiner's expression was expectant, friendly. "If you had to choose a single method for monitoring a burn patient during resuscitation, what would it be?"

My spirits lifted, my mind rallied. I replied with no hesitation: "Urinary output"

The friendly look disappeared. Before I could collect my thoughts, the next question was being asked. But I was no longer in that room at the Waldorf Astoria. I was spinning out of control, lost in another dimension.

I didn't recover until, as I now remember, Dr. Peacock was

standing beside me, putting his arm around my shoulder. "Great to see you this morning, Dr. Miller."

"Thank you . . ." was all I could manage, as I stepped backward, still facing his friendly grin.

He went on. "But you've got a lot of reading to do. You people who were trained at Brook Army want to drown those patients with Ringers Lactate." He took my hand firmly in his.

I nodded nervously, still taking small steps backward to the door which would lead to the hall – and safety.

"You of all people, after your time at Brook, should know better. *You have to pay attention to body weight!*" He exclaimed. "Keeping too much urine flowing overloads those patients . . . you just drown 'em. Well, maybe we can talk about it some other time."

Sweating now, I had almost reached the wall. Dr. Peacock still held my right hand in a firm grip; my left was searching blindly for the door knob I knew must be behind me.

"You have to be sure you don't create wet lungs," he continued. Then, release at last! – I found the door knob.

"Thank you," I gasped once more, as my left hand grasped the cool roundness of the brass knob.

In what seemed to me at the time a wonderful combination of good manners, coordination, and grace, I turned the knob, withdrew my right hand, turned and made a full stride through the door. My forward progress was abruptly halted by one of Peacock's sport coats.

"That, Dr. Miller, is the closet." His voice was expressionless.

I couldn't help blurting out, "The way things have been going this morning, maybe this is where I belong," and lunged for the real door to the hallway.

THE APPARITION

PROF DR. O. ONUR EROL ISTANBUL, TURKEY

Every man takes the limits of his own field
of vision for the limits of the world.
–Schopenhaver

In my clinic where I practice today, we paid very careful attention to the details of architecture and design. As a result of wanting a spacious office with lots of natural light, we have many skylights.

Recently, this gave quite a scare to the mother of one of our patients. While changing the bandages during a post surgery visit of a 19-year-old patient, he kept asking us, "Do you see the cat on the roof?" His mother thought her son had developed some kind of postsurgical schizophrenia and, as any mother would be, she became very concerned. She immediately asked the nurses if perhaps some medication or something from the operation was causing him to have hallucinations. When the patient heard his mother asking if her son had psychological problems, he became very disturbed and said, "Mom, what are you saying? Look up, you'll see a cat!" Because he was so insistent, everyone looked up and sure enough, there was a cat sitting on the skylight.

GRACE UNDER PRESSURE

WAYNE PERRON, M.D.   CALGARY, CANADA

The shemiehl lands on his back
and bruises his nose.
—Yiddish Proverb

A typical Thursday morning in the operating room. We had finished our first operation and were starting our second. The nurses brought the patient into the operating room. I finished marking the patient and the anesthetist started his anesthetic.

As was typical in a lot of operating rooms years ago, an autoclave was located within the operating room. This allowed for extra instruments or redoing of instruments between cases to speed up the process. On this particular day, the nurse loaded the autoclave and we were waiting for the instruments to sterilize. The anesthetist was carrying on with his usual regime of putting the patient to sleep, monitoring, making sure the lines were all open, etc.

We started the surgery on time. Unfortunately, two of our instruments had fallen on the floor and they had to be washed and placed in the sterilizer. We were able to carry on surgery comfortably without those instruments for the time being.

As we were operating, we heard a rumble coming from the sterilizer. It started as a small hiss, which indicated that the pressure was going up in the autoclave itself. This was followed by a very light rumble and then a sound that became quite menacing. We could not understand why this was happening. At one point, I looked at the anesthetist and could barely hear him talk. I started getting a little concerned at this point, as the intensity of the sound increased. Finally, I said "The autoclave is going to explode." All I could visualize was the massive autoclave door, weighing 200 lbs, flying across the room, picking me up midway and slamming me against the opposite wall. The anesthetist looked very concerned and hid behind the patient's bed. I quickly covered the patient up. Someone opened the door for the nurse to make a hasty retreat. Announcing there was a 911, the staff mobilized from the various parts of the operating room and assisted us in taking the patient across to another OR suite where she was quickly hooked up to monitors and another anesthetic machine. At no time was she in any danger. However, the noise continued. Our friendly in-house orderly, who had been around for years and knew pretty well everything about the functioning of the operating room, quickly appeared on the scene. After analyzing the situation, he walked into the operating room, turned the steam valve off and the horrendous sound of the exploding autoclave quickly ceased.

His only comment was, "If you idiots had closed the autoclave door tightly, there wouldn't have been any steam escape and you wouldn't have had this problem." We proceeded with our operation in another room and completed it successfully.

That particular operating room and autoclave were off bounds for several days. The maintenance people from the company came to inspect the autoclave and found it to be in perfect working order. Red faces and embarrassment were pretty common amongst the staff in the operating room the next day.

TAKE ME WITH YOU

RICHARD B. STARK, M.D.   NEW YORK, NY

> *The man who lives free from folly*
> *is not so wise as he thinks.*
> –La Rochefoucauld

As an international reconstructive plastic surgeon, I have seen a myriad of "before and after" emotional life stories that have brought cogent diplomacy to our country. One experience that lingers in my memory took place in the Dominican Republic. My host, an American-trained doctor, had scheduled the three lectures I was to give in the main hall of the autonomous university - well known as a political hot bed. But when we got there, we found to our dismay that it was being painted.

In the only other auditorium, a large group of the students was holding a political rally. My host interrupted, explaining that I would be lecturing there. We started to set up, only to find that the projection screen was full of holes. The alternative was an oblique white side wall which was plastered with political proclamations. The first one we took down and rolled up was a large pro-Castro poster. This met with a loud chorus of boos and catcalls. As angry students stormed out, one approached to within a few inches of my face and yelled, "What do you think you can teach us?" As he left, he scrawled on the wall, "YANKEE GO HOME."

"What an ominous beginning," I thought. These students were not only militantly anti-American, but more interested in politics than medicine Mao and Fidel - rather than rebuilding the face and parts of the body. Although we had expected several hundred, there were only a few dozen in the audience when I began.

My lecture was largely visual with projections of "before" pictures and enough operative views to show how the "after" result came about. The cases were of reconstructions of almost every external part of the body nose, ear, chin, cheek, breast, fingers, and by the time I came to the genital organs, I was aware of dark shapes quietly creeping in. When the lights went on, the hall was almost full.

Between the first and third lectures my host had arranged for me to perform three operations in the teaching hospitals for the residents to observe: The total reconstruction of the nose of a man who had lost it due to cancer; the repair in a single operation of a harelip and cleft palate, restoring speech to a teenage boy; and the removal from a man's leg of a crippling tumor that had been growing for seventeen years.

Evidently, word had spread that the Yankee Doctor did have something to teach. The third lecture, given to a standing room only audience, ended with prolonged applause and was followed by a question-and-answer period that went on for an hour. And to the graffiti on the wall, "YANKEE GO HOME," was added, "AND TAKE ME WITH YOU."

Well, I couldn't take him along, but indelibly imprinted in my memory were the before and after pictures of his face - hostile, flushed with anger in the beginning, and smiling, friendly at the end. That I did take along.

SMART TONGUE

FERDINAND OFODILE, M.D.
NEW YORK, NY

*A man is infinitely more complicated
than his thoughts.*
–Valery

In 1980, while I was a lecturer and consultant at the University of Ibadan, Nigeria, I received an urgent call that a four day old infant was being transferred on emergency basis to the university college hospital because of dysphagia and respiratory distress from a large mass in the tongue.

The child was brought to the emergency room by anxious parents in a taxi. Clinical examination revealed a 6x5 centimeter mass occupying two-thirds of the tongue. The child was dehydrated. The child was the second child of normal parents. After the initial examination, she was rehydrated and pertinent laboratory tests, including x-rays of the skull, facial bones and pharynx were done. All were normal. The mass was then excised in its entirety and the tongue was repaired. The specimen was sent for pathology examination.

To our great surprise the microscopic examination showed the mass to consist of pure brain tissue. As it turned out, it was the first case of pure brain ectopia in the tongue to be reported in the literature.

When we saw the child at follow-up and told the parents of our findings, they became hysterical. They wanted to know how the brain came about to grow in the tongue and whether, by removing it, we had effectively removed a vital functioning part of the child's brain. It took a lot of explaining, and the help of relatives, to calm them down and accept the fact that the child had not lost part of her brain.

BETTER BARTER

BERT BROMBERG, M.D.   MONTAUK, NY

*"Oh, what a tangled web we weave, when first we
practice to deceive!"*
–Sir Walter Scott

Our well-established plastic surgery group served a significant part of the community. After the fall of the Shah of
Iran, many wealthy Iranians migrated to the States and
particularly to our sphere of influence. I was well informed
regarding their trading skills and what I eventually experienced was the ultimate.

After successfully performing surgery on one of their clan,
the patient related to me the ardent desire of his mother to
undergo a facelift. Unfortunately, he related that she did not
have the necessary financial means. He wanted to know if I
would accept one of her Persian rugs as full or partial payment for the proposed surgery.

I turned the whole matter over to our office manager as a
sort of joke. After all, how could our ten member group par-
ticipate in the barter payment? Does one doctor get the
major design of the rug, one doctor the fringes and one the
periphery of the rug?

Well, to ease the calculus of the barter, we had the rug
appraised. Based on the appraisal, we told the patient that
we would accept the rug as partial payment and she would
be responsible for the balance. When I next saw her preop-
eratively, she proceeded to offer me a better deal.

Apparently, a man of my distinction and professional rank certainly deserved a much more valuable rug.

The newly proposed rug was of much greater value and was so clearly superior to the original rug, that I would now owe her the balance in cash, which amounted to several thousand dollars, prior to the surgery. A great scam, but obviously the deal fell through.

Beware of strangers bearing gifts, particularly Persian rugs!

POOR DIPLOMACY

WAYNE PERRON, M.D. CALGARY, CANADA

She had an unequaled gift of squeezing
big mistakes into small opportunities.
–Henry James

I was experiencing a typical day in the operating room. It was Friday afternoon and the operating room staff was slowing down. Everybody was readying for the weekend.

My day started as usual. On this particular Friday, I had a visitor from Japan. He was a plastic surgeon who wanted to watch a facelift. Having just arrived in Canada, he was jet lagged and looked a little weary. Since he could not speak English well, he brought a translator with him. We communicated well for the first hour. In the second hour, the procedure got a little mundane. The visitor said that he'd like to step out for some water and we told the translator where to take him. As is traditional in a lot of hospitals, the patient's bed is left outside the operating room for access when the procedure is finished. In our hospital, we had rather large hallways and the beds were pushed up against the wall just outside the door to the operating room. When the Japanese duo left the operating room, the translator went to get a glass of water. The surgeon, being somewhat tired, spotted this comfortable bed and laid down.

In our operating room, we had two orderlies that routinely worked so hard that it was mandatory that they take periodic rests throughout the day. Often, this would entail a small rest on one of the patient transfer beds outside the operating room. As it happened on this occasion, this position had been taken up by our physician guest and not by the orderly.

We have a very friendly operating room and the interaction between the staff was excellent. There was a lot of kidding and joking outside the operating room when the surgery was finished. This involved all of the staff. Dean, the orderly who was the glue in the operating room staff relations, was the fellow who took most of the rest breaks. The staff anesthetist, who was 6 ft 4, spotted an individual lying on the bed. Assuming it was Dean, he raised his arm and, with a very loud yelp, came down with this massive Karate chop that stopped just above the visiting surgeon's chest. By that time, the translator had come around the comer and witnessed this (apparent) act of aggression. Both the visiting surgeon and the translator were somewhat taken aback and, of course, the anesthetist was embarrassed to no end. The translator stuck his head into the operating room, said thank you very much for allowing us to observe the surgery, and then they quickly departed.

Chapter II

The Moving, the Touching, the Emotional

MIRSAD

ANTHONY WOLFE, M.D.   MIAMI, FL

In peace, sons bury their fathers; in war, fathers bury their sons.
—Herodotus

Mirsad, was his name – a nine-year-old Yugoslavian boy with a ruined face.

I came across him years ago, before the serious fighting had erupted in the Balkans. Someone in his country contacted me asking if I could help a young fellow who had sustained a gunshot injury to the face. I was sent x-rays and a photograph, and they revealed the extent of the destruction.

Although Mirsad had eyes, ears, a forehead, and a chin, the whole central part of his face, including the lips and nose, was nothing but a small pucker. The damage was so severe that I couldn't imagine how he could even eat in such a condition. Of course, I said that I would be glad to take care of him. The Yugoslavian government said that they would pay for his expenses.

When young Mirsad arrived with his father, he was wearing a surgical mask over his face to conceal the frankly hideous sight. The story was that a year or so earlier he had taken his father's hunting rifle down from a shelf. In doing so, he managed to drop it on the floor. The gun went off, and the hunting round entered his face under his chin, taking out the central part of his jaw, both lips, his nose, and part of his upper jaw.

I sent Mirsad over for preoperative photographs. While he was gone, I made arrangements for the first stage of the reconstructive work – removal of portions of the devitalized bone in the lower jaw, stabilization of the remaining segments of jaw with an external fixator, opening up the mouth, and opening up the nose-mouth orifice.

Our regular photographer was on vacation at that time, so we hired a substitute. When I went to check the preoperative pictures, I found to my horror that the idiot replacement cameraman had taken the photographs with the mask still on! Needless to say, our office quickly dissociated itself from this individual.

We went on to do a lot of work for Mirsad. This included reconstruction of the lower jaw, creation of new lips from tissue taken from his inner upper arm, rebuilding his palate using a transplanted muscle flap, opening up his nasal airways, reconstruction of the upper jaw using a bone graft from his hip, and eventually a new nose was built from forehead tissue.

At the end of all this, Mirsad looked presentable. There was certainly more work to be done. I was considering, for example, getting some bone-intergrated implants into both the upper and the lower jaw, so that he could be fitted with a dental prosthesis.

Money became an issue; the Yugoslavian government had provided only about $40,000, which was completely eaten up by his first hospitalization. But the Miami Children's Hospital came to the rescue and kindly agreed to allow me to continue operating on him until reconstruction was complete. When that point was reached, he would be able to return to his native Yugoslavia.

Mirsad and his father lived in an apartment provided by the hospital and stayed in Miami for over a year while surgery continued. I felt at that stage that it would be good for him to have some time without surgery. We planned to discharge him, at least temporarily, knowing that we could bring him back in a year or two to continue the work or perhaps arrange for the next stages to be handled by a European institution.

The boy had been "adopted" by a local motorcylcle club, and they laid on a big departure ceremony for him shortly before he set off for his homeland. He and his father were driven around the campus of the Children's Hospital on the backs of Harley Davidsons with the event being recorded by the television networks in Miami.

After this remarkable farewell, father and son flew back to Europe.

****

The postscript to this story is a tragic one:

About a month after their return home, Mirsad was playing in a group of Muslim children. A soldier, a man of the same nationality, but of a different religion, casually walked past and threw a hand grenade into their midst. Mirsad was killed.

Mirsad had been given the promise of a whole, functioning body and a fulfilling life. All that goodwill, all that energy, all wasted by an insane act of religious violence. We went from surgical triumph to mindless tragedy in little more than a year. We could do nothing but weep.

ENCOURAGEMENT FROM A MOTHER

D. MARCHAC, M.D.   PARIS, FRANCE

We wholly conquer only what we assimilate.
–Gide

My first major craniofacial case was a 19-year-old girl with a wide asymmetrical teleorbitism, associated with a distorted forehead and deviated nose. She was in good health and had a normal IQ.

The surgery was done in April 1971, with the help of a neurosurgeon and Francoise Firmin as assistant. It started at 9:00 a.m. and we finished at 2:00 a.m. the next day. The procedure was performed as planned, as I had seen Paul Tessier do many times: elevation of the frontal bone, removal of the excess bone on the midline, mobilization of the orbits and bringing them closer together, replacement of the frontal bone, correction of the asymmetry, reconstruction of the nose with a bone graft, canthopexies, elevation of the lateral lids, and, at that time, Z-plasty at the root of the nose to break the vertical midline scar.

Everything went well, and we were very pleased with the result. Three days later, she was back in the Plastic Surgery ward, doing fine, looking good, and I had the pleasure of presenting her to the staff during their rounds.

Two days later, the left side of her face started to swell. She developed a fever, became half-paralyzed, lost consciousness, and was transferred back to the neurosurgery ward. She died within 48 hours.

At the time, CT scans were not available, and x-rays and tomography did not show anything abnormal. The family refused an autopsy. It was assumed that she developed a thrombosis of the cranial veins, origination in the area of the left orbit.

I was devastated. The mother asked to see me. She had the same malformation as her daughter, an asymmetrical hypertelorism. Nevertheless, she had gotten married and had children. She told me that she had suffered all her life from her appearance and that she did not want her daughter to go through the same ordeal. She told me that I had warned her and her daughter of the risks, including the lethal one, and that they had accepted this risk. She added that she knew I had done all I could and that I should in no way get discouraged, that other patients would need my help!

Her words were of extraordinary importance to me. The head of the Plastic Surgery Unit, Professor Claude Dufourmentel, who had referred the patient to me, did not prevent me from continuing to perform this surgery. I learned years later that he called Paul Tessier about the matter and that Tessier had replied that it can happen, and that he thought I was well-trained and should continue.

I unfortunately experienced other disasters in my craniofacial career but never anything as dramatic as observed in that patient. And, each time, I thought of this admirable mother who had given me the courage not to give up.

RED SEA RESCUE

GHAITH F. SHUBAILAT, M.D.
AMMAN, JORDAN

Chance does nothing that has not been prepared beforehand.
   —De Tocqueville

August 1986: The headwaters of the Gulf of Aqaba were calm, and only a slight breeze softened the oppressive heat of the day. The Gulf is Jordan's link to the Red Sea, and a channel off the small resort town of Aqaba is set aside for speedboats and waterskis. Fifteen-year-old Zeid, accompanied by his two sisters and their friends, was enjoying the slow ride as he ran the engine of his father's new ski boat at a thousand revolutions a minute.

Thump.

The boat hesitated for a split second before continuing its passage through the sea. They all felt it. The passengers thought they had bumped into some small hunk of timber. But Zeid sensed instinctively that his craft had hit something alive – not a piece of flotsam.

He immediately looked astern and saw a struggling figure. He spun the wheel and reversed the boat's course. He came close to what he could now see as a drowning girl, the water around her stained red from the gushing blood of her injuries. Urgently, he shouted at his older sister, "Take over!" and pulled her to the wheel. In a matter of seconds, he was over the side, swimming frantically toward the girl whose struggles had now ceased.

Zeid realized that one of her arms was missing and that blood was pouring from other wounds. He managed to get her head out of the water and to hold it there, so at least she was not in imminent danger of drowning.

All this happened so quickly that he had no to time to think of what he would do next. He didn't have to – a boat manned by two professional sailors who had spotted the commotion while they were towing a skier closed from astern. They stopped their boat expertly next to the two figures in the water, and with the help of Zeid's other friends managed to pull them to safety. Not, however, before one of the ski-boat crewmen had fainted at the sight of the bloody wreckage of the girl's body and its missing arm.

The rescuers transferred Zeid back to his own boat, then with the girl on board headed at high speed for the beach, saying that they would get her to the hospital as fast as they could. Zeid revved up his engine, running-in procedure abandoned in the urgency of the moment, and roared the planting boat back to the beach in front of the family's vacation house.

Breathless and frantic, Zeid ran to his father.

"Dad, I hit a swimmer. Her arm was severed. She's on her way to the hospital. Please rush to help her. I'm going back to find the arm."

Zeid's father, Dr. Ghaith Shubailat, knew that his son was competent to attempt what he was setting out to do, although he doubted if he'd be successful. He also knew that he had to get to the small field hospital in Aqaba to do what he could to help the badly injured girl. No one could have been better qualified than Dr. Shubailat. Just two years earlier, he had retired from a full military career in the Royal Medical Services of the Jordanian Armed Services. His early medical training was in London, after which he became a general surgeon and then finally completed his residency in plastic surgery at Georgetown University in Washington, D.C. In the 1970s and the 1980s, he headed up a program of training top-class plastic surgeons in Jordan and became a leader in the introduction of microsurgery into the military service – a first in the Arab world. Press and television media had given wide coverage to his microvascular replantation of severed limbs and on the handling, cooling, and transport of amputated body parts.

Dr. Shubailat rushed to the simple hospital and arrived just as the critically damaged girl was being wheeled into the emergency room. He took over examination and immediately saw that she had a complete amputation of the left arm just below the shoulder, as well as multiple open chest wounds, superficial abdominal wounds, and left thigh wounds. In a macabre contrast to her tenuous hold on life, she was still wearing her snorkel mask and tube.

The doctor found that the surgical residents in charge were young interns he had helped train in general surgery at Amman's King Hussein Medical Center. The anesthesiologist was a second-year resident – his superior was away on vacation. So the team was not what he would have called highly experienced.

The patient was resuscitated and taken to the operating theater. Dr. Shubailat put in a chest tube, closed the multiple wounds, and then waited for news of recovery of the severed limb. He looked around him to see what was available for the surgery he would have to perform. He mentally noted some ophthalmic instruments, a couple of vascular clamps, and a few marrow nails. There was no operating microscope, and he did not have his loupes with him. He was in a simple hospital with only basic equipment. His thoughts raced ahead to how he would tackle the complex task of reattaching the arm, if and when it was recovered.

But back at the beach, Zeid found two Coast Guard divers patrolling in their boat. He hailed them frantically, and they swung around to where he was shouting from the shore. Breathless, he told them what had happened; within minutes, they were at the scene of the accident.

One of the divers immediately back-flipped over the side, and with good fortune found the arm lying on the sand in twenty-five feet of water. He brought it to the surface, and commandeered the icebox of a nearby pleasure craft. Carefully the arm was placed on the ice (the doctor's television programs must have made an impression!) and the dive boat raced back to the beach with its precious cargo.

Zeid rushed to his father with the precious icebox – the time the arm had been without blood supply would have been about an hour. The doctor went straight to work. He rejoined the bones with narrow nails and reconnected the severed arm artery. Less than two hours after the damage had been done, blood was once again flowing into the reattached limb.

This first and most vital step had been accomplished. But the doctor could not reconnect the smaller veins, as the injury site was so badly torn up. He began the long and difficult task of bridging the veins with grafts – much more difficult because the hospital's equipment was so limited.

But one essential resource was instantly available.

Blood.

As news of the accident spread around the town, a crowd of some three hundred people – seamen, fishermen, shopkeepers, port workers – gathered around the hospital, all offering to donate blood. The spirit of helpfulness in this community of simple folk gave a huge boost to the morale of the small surgical team fighting to save not only the girl's limb, but her very life. The young corporal lab technician working alone crossmatched and prepared 250 units of blood in three nonstop days. By the end of it, the patient had received forty units without a single adverse reaction.

Through his senior status in the medical services of the Jordanian military, Dr. Shubailat had become a friend of the late King Hussein and his wife, Queen Noor. It so happened that the royal couple was also vacationing in Aqaba, where they were neighbors. Six hours after the emergency surgery started, the king telephoned to ask for news of the patient.

The doctor explained that the patient could not be moved, and certainly not evacuated by air, because the tiny rejoined veins kept blocking, requiring surgical intervention within minutes to redo the vein repairs to change grafts. The king immediately ordered his executive jet to fly to the capital, Amman, some two hundred miles to the north, as many times as it was needed, to bring everything the doctor required for successful continuation of the surgery. In came his loupes, his microsurgical instruments, suture material, doctors who had been his plastic surgery students in his

Army days, his scrub nurse, and a relief for his exhausted anesthesiologist.

The king cancelled all of his appointments and stayed in Aqaba for three days in support of his friend. He understood that medical history was being written in Jordan. He wanted to be sure that this attempt in a small provincial field hospital to reattach a severed limb lost in the Red Sea would succeed. He knew that a wonderful and loyal medical team was pulling out all stops. He also knew that emotional support was coming not only from the local community but from the whole nation, galvanized by these dramatic days.

Jordan is a country where tribal and family feelings still run strong. Emotions can be strained to breaking point by the sort of near-tragedy which had just occurred. Here, King Hussein played a key role. During a brief lull between surgical procedures, he called the doctor and the father of the fifteen-year-old victim (whose name was Hanada) together. The two men knew each other well: Hanada's father had retired as Police Chief of Aqaba, where his daughter had learned to swim and dive. The king spoke,

"Hanada is my daughter, and Zeid is my son. I want you both to shake hands, and then all of us will help Dr. Ghaith to go back and continue his work."

With the way ahead cleared of potential antagonisms, the work indeed continued. During the next three days and nights, the surgeon operated for a total of 30 hours, regrafting veins. On day four the patient was stable enough to be flown by helicopter, accompanied by the surgeon, to the King Hussein Medical Center in Amman. Here, a whole month was spent reopening thrombosed veins until there was enough blood circulation to support the limb.

In the following year, the doctor carried out no less than twenty-five reconstructive procedures, many of them with baffling technical terms but very successful outcomes – latissimus dorsi myocutaneous flap, serratus anterior microvascular free flap, plating and bone grafting the humerus, nerve repairs, sural nerve graft to ulnar nerve, tissue expanders, and multiple revisions of scars. His final "parting gift," five years after the accident, was rhinoplasty to enhance the look of her nose.

Hanada's left arm made a good recovery. Not a hundred percent, but she has developed movements that disguise any remaining deficiency. She cannot play the piano, but she got her BA degree in English Literature, and is in good employment.

Zeid went on to college in the United States and graduated from the Citadel in Charleston, South Carolina, with a degree in Computer Science. He then took a Master's in Health Administration from the University of South Carolina, and is now a senior consultant with Microsoft in New York.

CHU

MARK GORNEY, M.D.   NAPA, CA

*The world is neither wise nor just, but it makes up for all its folly
by being damnable sentimental.*
–T. H. Huxley

"Psychic income" is a phrase we in the medical profession
sometimes use – not without a touch of cynicism – to
describe the reward which replaces money where charitable
surgery is concerned. On very rare occasions, however, that
callused shell of emotional indifference with which we protect ourselves is breached.

An event thirty-odd years ago was one of those occasions.
War-torn Vietnam provided enough horrific injury, inde-
scribable pain, and sheer misery to fill one's memory bank to
overflowing. We, in the medical teams which worked to alleviate the results of man's inhumanity to man, were front-
line participants in, and witnesses of, this dreadfulness.
And yet we almost always managed to maintain our professional distance. To have done otherwise would not have
helped us; and, by lessening our objectivity, would certainly
not have helped our patients.

Almost always. But not that day in the Barsky Unit in
Vietnam.

In Dong Hospital was a charitable house that represented
what passed for a children's hospital in Saigon. An English
nurse from Ni Dong called one morning to tell us that they

were looking after a pathetic nine-year-old fragment of humanity, dying slowly and painfully from extensive unhealed burns. Would you please take him?

We agreed to do so. But when he arrived at the Unit, we wondered why we had. He weighed just forty-one pounds, a ravaged specter of a child, skin stretched taut over his skeletal face. His arms and legs were mere pipestems, covered with foul-smelling, yellowish green rags which we had come to associate with transferred burns in Vietnam.

His hold on life was clearly tenuous. But he had one feature which burned itself into my memory. His eyes. Whether from high fever or from a fathomless rage to live, they glittered black and tear-rimmed from sunken sockets.

We found out only two things about him. His name was Chu; and he had been brought to Saigon from somewhere near Pleiku, the scene of heavy fighting and the use of a lot of napalm.

The staff at Ni Dong thought that he was the only survivor of his family. Artillery shells and rockets had hit their village, and he suffered third-degree burns over sixty percent of his body. At some point a botched attempt to put skin grafts on him had been made. Not only had the grafts failed; because of his advanced stage of malnutrition, the donor sites had not healed. The raw granulation tissue was salmon pink and had the consistency of jelly. His dressings were crawling with maggots.

We had no idea how long he had been in this state.

Over the next few days, Chu was tubbed in a whirlpool tank, received blood transfusions, and his dressings were replaced.

The change in his appearance was near miraculous. His skin turned from dung-colored to bronze. He started eating, and after a week the sharp outline of his rib cage visibly softened. He even managed a weak smile when coaxed.

We got hold of some chocolate for him. This was something he had never tasted, and he ate it ravenously. Our pediatrician built him a model airplane, which immediately became his most prized possession.

We took two weeks of gradual preparation to get him ready for surgery. During that waiting period, the nurses asked about his family. He found it impossible to talk about them directly, but putting two and two together we concluded that they were all dead. With one possible exception: his father, who had been outside their dwelling when it was attacked.

Over the next few weeks, Chu underwent surgery four times. The days between operations were filled with undiluted agony. Even with the most tender care, each dressing change was like being filleted alive. As any child would, he cried while he was being greatly hurt, but he gritted his teeth and clenched his hands on the side-rails until his nails cut into his palms. The pain was intolerable.

After what seemed an eternity, his wounds healed, his arms and legs began to get some flesh on the bones. But the edges of the grafts were still purple welts, and he found movement difficult. In spite of this, we saw him being propelled around the hallways in his wheelchair, playing with his precious airplane. We all felt uplifted and excited by these improvements, gained at such a price.

But the unspoken question hung in the air: "What next?"

The same English nurse who had brought Chu to us originally came in to see him. She was amazed and deeply
moved to see him now. She told us that there was a story
currently on the Vietnam grapevine that an old gentleman
had been searching for his son in the Saigon hospitals,
believing that he might still be alive.

By coincidence, one of our nurses had a boyfriend in the military, serving at that time in the Pleiku area. She sent a
message explaining the situation, in the faint hope that he
might have some information. A few days later, the English
nurse called again, and gave us the news – rather tentatively,
not wishing to raise false hopes – that a little man had
shown up at Ni Dong with a torn, faded picture of a child
much younger than Chu. It was just possible . . . .

We asked her to bring him over, and we put the child in a
wheelchair, hair combed, face scrubbed. No one told him
why this was going on. He was taken downstairs and
parked outside the building under a bronze plaque which
reads: "IT IS BETTER TO LIGHT ONE CANDLE THAN
CURSE THE DARKNESS." Some of the nurses who had
given so much of themselves to bring him back into the light
of life came downstairs too.

A Volkswagen turned into the area in front of the unit and
stopped by the entrance. An old man – classic Vietnamese
peasant face, grizzled and worn, wispy beard, topped by the
usual conical hat – was helped from the car, some thirty feet
from the nurses grouped around the wheelchair. He
appeared to be totally confused, lost. He stood slightly bent,
rooted to the spot, searching faces uncomprehendingly.

Suddenly, the boy saw who he was. He let out a long, shriek-
ing wail. He began to rock back and forth in his wheelchair,

not attempting to get out. Rhythmically back and forth, back and forth, wailing and screaming in Vietnamese between contorted gasps.

As understanding dawned, the old man seemed to collapse as his knees suddenly buckled. The English nurse ran toward him, but he was neither sick nor hurt. He fell to his knees, forehead to the ground, palms flat in front of him. He wailed also, raised his head, and then bent down again to touch head and hands on the concrete. Up and down, up and down, tears coursing down that leathery face, while the rest of us froze into a tableau in the heat and humidity of that Vietnamese day.

Neither father nor son made any attempt to move toward each other. Some of the nurses tried to urge the old man to stand up, but all he did was to grasp their ankles and try to kiss their feet. The boy shrieked and rocked – back and forth, scream! back and forth, scream! – until a nurse wheeled him to his father, still on his knees on the hard driveway.

The old man stayed kneeling and embraced the boy. He stroked his hair. Father and son rocked back and forth, together now, crying and wailing in eerie unison.

The emotional wall between the team and their patient was broken now, broken into fragments. The professional reserve of the group who had gathered under the BETTER TO LIGHT ONE CANDLE sign was blown away by the intense emotion of that reunion. Totally out of control, they ran, sobbing, back into the building.

MORALITY AND MORTALITY

MARK GORNEY, M.D.   NAPA, CA
TERRY R. KNAPP, M.D.   LONGMONT, CO

In utrumque paratus
Seu versare dolos seu certae occumberre morti.
–Virgil

This is really two stories. The first relates directly to plastic surgery, the third world, and the tragedy of a child's mortality. The second paints a picture of collision – collision between medicine, morality, and the law.

Virgil had it right: "Prepared for either event, to set his traps or to meet with certain death." Death was the keynote of the child's life in the first tale, the setting of traps, at least in a legal sense, the essence of the second.

A great chasm separates medicine and the law. Practitioners of law are trained to see life as conflict; the adversarial nature of our legal system precludes any other philosophy. And for legal conflict, we need resolution, winners, and losers. Because of this need, lawyers find it neither logical nor convenient to accept that the process of living brings events over which no one has any control.

Medical practitioners, conversely, are trained to accept the idea that life is a game of chance, that it has a beginning and an end, and that although we have a limited measure of control over when it begins, we have very little control over when – or how – it ends. All that we humans can do at the point when the body falters and fails is to fall back on the beliefs of fate, destiny, philosophy, or religion.

It is difficult for patients to accept that an unfavorable outcome, whatever form the treatment may take, can be truly inevitable. Combining these thought processes – unwillingness to consider the uncertainties of life, and the concept that all events are the result of win/lose situations – it is not surprising that our society has drifted comfortably into the uniquely American concept that for every bad thing that happens, someone has to pay.

The media swamp us with misconceptions about the limitations of medical technology and the possibility of "miracle cures." Why then would anyone not assume that if something goes wrong it must be someone else's fault? The old Hippocratic dictum "above all, do no harm" has metamorphosed into "above all, prevent any harm from ever occurring – or else!"

The medical/legal chasm opens up widest in the context of a lawsuit involving alleged medical malpractice or negligence. The plaintiff has the philosophical mind-set of our time, the mind-set that all outcomes must be favorable; this reinforces the training and conditioning of the attorney which leads him to identify the winners and act against the losers. The attorney who defends a doctor against these accusations would define the issue as maximum social irresponsibility.

Against this background, then, think about these two short tales. One concerns itself with mortality, and its acceptance in a third world context. The other can be considered as more of a morality tale, the battle between winner and loser, between responsibility and irresponsibility, and perhaps between right and wrong, in today's America.

INTERPLAST is a surgical organization from Stanford University that provides charitable reconstructive surgery services to third-world countries. Besides myself, Terry Knapp, the Latin American team includes the leader, Don Laub, professor, program director, and founder of INTER-PLAST; Harry Hatzel, senior pediatrician at the Palo Alto Clinic; the top anesthesiologist from the Stanford heart team, Kent Garman; and Lorne Eltherington. All have vast experience in this type of work.

At our clinic in a Latin American country one Friday, we evaluated a nine-month-old boy, Salvador. He had been born with a wide-open bilateral cleft lip and palate defect. He was the fifth child of a devoted but dirt-poor peasant couple in their late thirties.

We had seen him on previous visits since soon after his birth. He had failed to thrive; he was underweight, could not suckle, and was extremely difficult to feed – which of course was part of the problem. Until this visit, he had not come up to the classic "rule of 10s" criteria for surgery.

This time, however, he weighed a shade over ten pounds, and his hemoglobin was just over ten also. Our pediatrician felt that the child met the criteria and saw no apparent reason to postpone. The anesthesiologists carried out their own examination and concurred with this conclusion. To the parent's delight, he was scheduled for that Saturday morning.

Although I was still in residency, this was my sixth INTER-PLAST trip, and Don Laub had put me in charge of administering this particular program. Because of my experience, I was to be the operator, with the Chief assisting and supervising. Everything started normally. We made our incisions and proceeded with the dissection of flaps quite uneventfully for about thirty minutes. There was insignificant blood loss, but we suddenly noticed that the slight ooze had turned quite dark. Almost simultaneously, we sensed a commotion behind the screen. Anesthesia said, "Stop a minute. We have a problem."

In an instant, all drapes and covers were off. All of us, including the pediatrician, who had just come in, worked frantically for an hour and a half to save this child. Cardiac monitor tracking showed that his heart was in agonal rhythm, but no clear-cut arrhythmia could be seen. His heart just quit. No amount of stimulation – chemical, mechanical, or electrical – could bring him back.

Salvador had quite simply died on the table.

It would be an understatement to say that we were shattered and heartbroken – for the baby, for his family, for the INTERPLAST program, for our host, and for our own inability to recover the child. Anxiety and remorse lay over the team like a thick fog. Don Laub was shaken to the core. Four years of success and overcoming all kinds of difficulties, and now this, the first time we had ever lost a patient.

I was asked to supervise the cleanup while the others went to find the hospital director, the priest, and the family. I looked at Salvador, as he was about to be wrapped in a plastic sheet for the morgue. His face, the focus of our effort, was a ghastly mess. He looked as though a hand grenade had exploded right in front of his nose. There was dried blood everywhere, devastated tissues cut apart. His appearance was far worse than the deformity with which he had entered the operating room.

I asked the nurse to lay him back on the table, and leave me alone with him for about forty-five minutes. Then she left, shutting the door behind her. I cleaned him up and finished repairing his lip as meticulously as I knew how. The thought crossed my mind that – had he lived – I would have been proud to show him off at rounds the next morning. I called the staff back in, they wrapped him up again, and with a lump in my throat I watched them trundle him to the the morgue.

An hour or so later, Don Laub returned. He looked ashen as he said, "We finally found the parents. They'll be here tomorrow." There was much crying and mutual hugging, and then we all left the clinic with little in the way of questions or conversation. The evening passed in the deepest gloom. Our local hosts were worried about possible repercussions, both political and social, and about the future of the program. Traditionally, our team would have gathered for stress-relieving drinks and dinner, music, and laughter. That night, we did nothing except to take up a collection for a small wooden coffin.

The next morning, the Sunday, the team drove to the hospital to pack up and go home. As we pulled into the driveway, we saw a group of people gathered in front of the doors. Among them were Salvador's parents. We got out of the car, dreading the ugly scene we felt was inevitable.

The father left the group and approached us. He asked hesitantly – in Spanish, of course – if he could speak with the head doctor. Don nodded his agreement, and the father turned and gestured for his wife and the priest to come forward.

The message from the parents was simple and straightforward. There was no mistaking the father's meaning, even though he spoke through pain and tears. It hit our hearts like a sledgehammer.

"We want to thank you and your team for everything you did for our little son. That he is now dead is God's will. But thanks to all of you, he can now go through eternity in heaven, and meet God with a normal face and a beautiful smile.

Muchos gracias!"

* * * * * * * * *

Jeremy, a young and successful industrial designer was disconcerted and then frightened by a whole spectrum of bizarre symptoms. He consulted his physician, a highly respected specialist, who examined him thoroughly.

"I cannot immediately make a fully accurate diagnosis, so we'll need to do a number of tests. Among those tests I recommend that we include one for HIV. Unlikely of course, but I'd like to rule every possibility out."

Blood was drawn, a urine sample taken, and the doctor ordered a number of tests from the lab, among them the specified HIV. Just in case.

When the telephone call came through to his office to say the HIV test was positive, Jeremy went into a state indistinguishable from physical shock. He was unable to work, his inventive and creative capabilities hibernated, a cold horror gripped his mind. The specter of full-blown AIDS dominated his outlook.

In a matter of days this initial shock gave way to a longer-term depression. Even this, however, gradually left him, and he found once more the ability to think. He reasoned that because his life span would certainly be severely curtailed by this insidious virus, he should leave his profession and devote himself to doing the things and seeing the sights that he'd missed during his hard climb to success.

From an outsider's objective viewpoint, the question could be raised – why did he not ask for the test to be repeated, to either confirm or deny his status? The answer seems to lie in his having had an isolated homosexual encounter in his recent past, making him reluctant to the point of inaction to pursue the issue.

His mind made up, he decided to travel the world. He closed his studio, sold his belongings and condominium, severed all his relationships, and took off, leaving no forwarding address.

After a few months of international travel, his strange original symptoms slowly released their hold on him, and he began to feel quite normal. But he did not change his mind or his new way of life; he knew that this was not unusual after a positive HIV diagnosis.

Eight months after he had left America, Jeremy found himself in Paris. There he had made some new friends, who persuaded him to arrange a consultation with one of the world's experts in AIDS. This physician, not unnaturally, had him re-tested – twice – and each time the result came back negative.

The evening after he heard the results, he went on a champagne binge which left him with the mother of all hangovers. When this wore off, he caught the next flight home and immediately confronted his doctor. The test was again repeated, and again proved negative.

Why would this have been? The only possible explanation is that there must have been misidentification of the original specimen, but it would be impossible to determine who was responsible, the physician's staff or the laboratory. Both see large numbers of similar cases, and a microscopically small amount of error creeps in. Jeremy filed suit against both, on the grounds of negligence and extreme emotional distress. He also sought punitive damages.

The case went to trial, where the jury learned that Jeremy was not only still healthy, but wealthy as well. The defense argued that the plaintiff had in essence merely been driven to take a long-postponed sabbatical and that damages, if any, should be strictly limited because during any sabbatical he would have earned nothing.

The jury bought this line of argument, awarding him a nominal sum for negligence. However, the money he received for "emotional distress" ran into seven figures.

JENNY

STEPHAN ARIYAN, M.D.   NEW HAVEN, CT

"...The greatest mistake you make in life
is to be continually fearing you will make one."
—E. Hubbard

Jenny was just eight years old when she suffered severe burn injuries to her entire body. When I treated her, she had ninety percent full-thickness burns, and there was little hope that she would survive.

However, miraculously, she did survive, even though she had to have skin grafts all over her body taken from the remaining areas that had not been burned. Eventually, she recuperated well, and her subsequent upbringing was taken on by her grandparents.

Later, she came back to me for the creation of a thumb/index finger web space – both her hands had "cocooned" as the result of the loss of her fingers. The operation was a success. She mastered the art of using a pencil and even developed the ability to tie her shoe laces with only this web space.

Jenny had dreamed for a long time of going to a Caribbean beach, and at last the dream came true. A nonprofit group operating in the state aimed to fulfill the wishes of children with chronic or terminal illnesses. These good people heard of Jenny's wish and made arrangements for her to make the trip with her grandparents.

The family arrived at the resort, and soon the young girl was enjoying the fun of poolside in the idyllic island climate. It wasn't long before she saw at the far end of the pool one of the local craftsmen giving basket-weaving lessons to adults and children, one of the educational activities arranged by the hotel. She asked to be included, and the grandparents signed her up for the course the very next day.

Jenny arrived for the lesson. The instructor was startled to see the girl with her burned features, no hair, and missing fingers. He was very concerned about her. He spotted the grandparents at the other end of the pool, walked over to them, and upbraided them for putting her into the course.

"I cannot understand why you would sign her up." The man's voice was laced with anger. "She will be completely frustrated trying to weave baskets from palm leaves. It is obvious that this will be impossible for her."

The grandparents looked at each other, smiled, and gently suggested to the teacher that he not judge Jenny so quickly.

"At least give her a chance to take advantage of her lessons," the grandfather added. "Perhaps you might both learn something."

Reluctantly, the instructor agreed. Jenny then demonstrated to him and to the other participants just how skillful she had become with her damaged hands as she had grown. She soon mastered the task. The session ended with her very successful weaving of a basket, and with the instructor's transition from concern to admiration.

After the family had returned home, Jenny came to see me for one of her office visits. She was shining with pride as she told me the story and gave me the basket as a gift.

To this day, that basket still sits with pride on my office credenza.

Chapter III

Patients' Attitudes

ALWAYS LISTEN TO YOUR MOTHER

RICHARD LEVINE, M.D.   SAN ANTONIO, TX

Problems cannot be solved at the same
awareness that created them.
–Albert Einstein

This story reflects on the human nature and as the frustrating aspect of being disappointed by the moral character of our patients. I was called to see a patient with a mediastinal abscess after open-heart surgery. It was clear this patient had a mycotic aneurysm and was on his deathbed. The heart surgeon and I decided that a "hail Mary" approach was necessary, and we discussed with the patient's family the potential and likely outcome. The deftly skilled heart surgeon opened the sternum, released the mycotic aneurysm and only a Foley catheter kept us from exsanguination.

The segment of the aorta was necrotic and needed to be replaced, but in the face of infection, a prosthetic device was out of the question. We took out a rib and rotated a pectoralis flap and wrapped the aorta in the pectoralis flap. This patient survived and did well postoperatively.

Six months later, a malpractice suit was filed against the heart surgeon and myself. It turns out the patient had forgotten that he had been to the emergency room with chest pain at some point in his past and so his insurance company declined to pay for his open heart surgery and the treatment of complications. Of course, in lawyer language, that meant let's sue somebody, and we were the likely targets.

90

The rest of the story is as interesting. My malpractice carrier told me not to get involved with any issues, not to speak with the attorney, and not to speak with the patient. I took it upon myself to call the patient's mother with whom I had sat in the recovery room and spent quite a lot of time in the postoperative period. When she found out that her son had filed suit against us, she made him drop the suit and send me a letter of apology. To this day, I get a Christmas card from her every year.

PLASTIC SURGERY AND DANCE

CHRISTINE M. RODGERS, M.D.
DENVER, CO

. . . clear dances done in the sight of heaven.
–Richard Purdy Wilbur

Dance and plastic surgery are two disciplines which do not immediately come to mind as being linked. In my practice, however, I have found that many of my patients have taken to dancing as a beneficial part of their post-surgery rehabilitation, physically and psychologically.

Dance has always been an important thread in my life's fabric. I started with ballet lessons at the tender age of five. I have continued dancing up to the present day and plan to go on, at least as much as I can without interfering with my primary responsibilities as a surgeon. In my general and plastic surgery residencies, I went on with my dancing, although some of my professors took a dim view of the activity; they took the view that such outside interests indicated less than full dedication on the doctor's part.

Far from it. Dance has integrated well with my profession, and it has helped me as well as others.

During my career in plastic surgery, I found the principle of integrating dance with medicine was able, in many cases, to help the healing process by creating in patients a more optimistic attitude. When I came across patients who were more than usually troubled or upset, I took them with me to a dance class; they invariably developed a better body image and a more robust mental outlook on their disease.

Suzanne was a case in point. When she returned home from the hospital after a mastectomy, she was confronted with the shattering fact that her husband had changed the locks on all the doors. He had decided that her breast cancer was unacceptable to him. He did not want to deal with it and, of course, wanted no more of his wife.

Unsurprisingly, Suzanne's self-esteem dropped to zero. She lost all sense of her own worth, and these negative feelings resulted in her gaining 180 pounds in weight.

It took eight years before she came to me to talk about getting rid of some of the excess fat she had out on, and about reconstruction of her missing breast, using some abdominal fat. We went ahead with the procedures and, during her recuperation, we became good friends. I persuaded her to come with me to jazz and ballet classes. Although dance itself did not greatly interest her, the experience led her take up tai chi, the gentle Chinese art of slow exercise movements, which she found more in tune with her personality.

Net result: Suzanne's self-image improved dramatically and, after all those years, she found herself able to mix socially without feeling ashamed of her body. Dance itself had not brought about these changes; but, in combination with plastic surgery, it had led to a lifestyle of normality and optimism.

My many experiences of this type led me into increasing involvement with dance and its interface with the practice of medicine. In the 1990s I took more classes and joined a contemporary dance company in Denver. Together with Thomas Dixon, a professional dancer and wonderfully kind teacher, I started a dance class for breast cancer survivors. We combined jazz, African, funk, and modern and lyrical jazz. Thomas's genius was to make all my patients feel as though they were hearing the applause of an enthusiastic audience on a Broadway stage.

The women who came to the class felt free. Wigs came off – they had no need to hide their bald but beautiful heads. The group felt as though they were sisters and friends, and the spirit of the dance revealed the little girl hiding in each of us. Even though we were not a breast cancer patient support group, talk often veered round to who was in therapy, who had a setback, whose hair was coming back. But this was not the purpose and function of the group, which was to move to music with unfrozen limbs, to be lithe and limber, and to feel good about just who one was.

HOW A DISFIGUREMENT CAN HELP

D. MARCHAC, M.D.   PARIS, FRANCE

The same fire purifies gold and consumes straw.
–Italian Proverb

A young boy of 18 from a West African country was sent to me for a facial neurofibromatosis – Elephant Man Disease. His left eyelid, nose, and cheek were distorted by the disease.

I removed the lesion in stages and, in between the operations, instead of going back to Africa, he stayed in Paris and went to school. He finished his junior high school and started to study economics at the university. His country's embassy was paying his living expenses, and the university is free in France, so he could manage all that quite well and was doing fine.

After 18 months and three operations, I told him that I thought we had to stop, that I could no longer significantly improve his appearance. His nose and cheeks were practically normal. He still had some irregularities at the eyelid level, but they were easily hidden by sunglasses.

He then explained to me that he needed another year to finish his studies and begged me to plan more surgeries so he could stay in France. I agreed to that, drew up a certificate, and did some more touch-ups.

I recently visited his country for a PSEF meeting and I met him. He became a high-ranking state civil servant, the Director of Development in the north of the country. He was wearing a dark suit, white shirt and tie, and looked great. With his sunglasses, one does not notice anything special. He was happily married and had nice kids.

He told me that since he was not of the same ethnic group as the president of his country, he would have had no chance to go to the university there. He explained that it was only because of his illness that he had been sent to France and was able to obtain a university degree. This man considered himself fortunate – for him, his disfiguring disease had been a blessing in disguise!

MY TURN

GARRY S. BRODY, M.D.   LOS ANGELES, CA

*There is more felicity in the far side
of baldness than young men can
possibly imagine.*
–L.P. Smith

Early in my practice, a 62-year-old gentleman consulted me concerning rhinoplasty. He looked very much like Ed Asner, and I guess I betrayed my skepticism until he offered the following explanation: He had always hated his nose, but he had four children, all of whom he had to put through college. For the last 10 years, he had an invalid wife who consumed all of his time and most of his resources. She had passed away, the children had all graduated, and so he said to me, "Now it's my turn!"

AVOIDING PAIN

HILTON BECKER, M.D.   BOCA RATON, FL

It is always the secure who are humble.
–Chester

One day, I was getting ready to do a local procedure on a patient and, as I raised the syringe to infiltrate the local anesthesia, the patient said to me, "Now, we are not going to hurt each other, are we doctor?" I proceeded to inject the local anesthetic as slowly and as painlessly as possible.

THE DONKEY

JACOB GOLAN, M.D.
JERUSALEM, ISRAEL

I don't want to be the cheese,
I just want to get out of the trap.
–Spanish Proverb

Before the present situation in and around Israel, life was much quieter. We used to get many patients from the Arab cities and towns nearby.

One such was a man who was brought into the emergency room with a most unusual injury. He had been bitten by a donkey! Now, as a rule, donkeys are the most docile of animals and reasonably intelligent, but his attacker was the exception that proved the rule.

I went to the ER to examine the man. He must have been some fifty years of age. His nose and upper lip were missing, having been taken off by the suddenly aggressive animal.

He had gone that morning to the market of Nablos, where he had bought the donkey. He tied a rope around its neck – a common practice in that region – and started to lead the beast back to his village.

On the way, the donkey saw a beautiful she-donkey standing by the side of the road. He evidently liked the look of her; for, when the villager stopped for a few minutes, persistent tugging on the rope indicated that he wanted to pursue a love affair more actively. The man, anxious to move on, pulled on the rope to move his new donkey away.

This made the donkey angry. Without hesitation, he opened his mouth wide and bit his new master's face with enough force to remove his nose and lip.

Local people saw what was happening and took the injured man to the hospital in Nablos, which had no experience in the type of surgery required. They sent him on to us.

It took us some weeks to restore his lip and nose, but eventually he was back to almost his normal state. He was so grateful for the treatment that he'd received, he would stop by once in a while to visit our hospital and to show us his beautiful renewed face. Such visits came to an end, not surprisingly, when the political situation worsened, and we never saw him again.

We just hope that the lesson was sharp enough to teach him to be more careful with his donkeys from then on.

CAN'T GET NO SATISFACTION

HILTON BECKER, M.D.   BOCA RATON, FL

The girl who can't dance, says the band can't play.
—Yiddish Proverb

I've always been impressed by how grateful breast reconstruction patients are, even if the results are suboptimal. There was one exception to this rule. That was an elderly patient who I thought was a little too old to have a breast reconstruction done; but, nevertheless, she wanted to have it done. She ended up getting a superb result and decided to proceed with nipple-areola reconstruction. She was happy all along until she came back for the six-month follow-up, at which she answered, "I really like the breasts, but I'm very disappointed that my nipple does not become erect."

MRS. DORIAN GREY

BRUCE ACHAUER, M.D. ORANGE, CA

The hours of folly are measured by the clock;
but of wisdom, no clock can measure.
—Blake

Another patient in her early 70s had a dramatic improvement by eliminating a baggy chin and neckline, deep nasolabial fold lines, and heavy eyelids with bags under the eyes. She was thrilled and could scarcely wait to show off her new look on a visit to her native New York and all the relatives there. When we asked about the relatives' reaction to her new appearance, she said they were unimpressed. This seemed like an inappropriate reaction, and so we inquired how she could account for their non-reaction.

"That's easy," she said. "I haven't been back for a visit for 20 years, so I look now just the way they remembered me, 20 years ago!" Needless to say, she didn't mind at all that her relatives didn't appreciate the change.

UNFORESEEN CONSEQUENCES

JACOB GOLAN, M.D.   JERUSALEM, ISRAEL

*Men stumble over the truth from time to time, but
most pick themselves up and hurry off as if
nothing happened.*
–Sir Winston Churchill

Occasionally, the practice of cosmetic surgery can lead to entirely unexpected outcomes.

A lady of forty-something years came to see me one day to ask to be considered for breast augmentation surgery. She was the wife of a rich man who was a well-known figure in Jerusalem and mother of his four daughters. I examined her and found her to be a suitable candidate for the procedure. I performed the operation, which went without incident; and, after a brief recovery period, she was more than pleased with the results.

We scheduled regular follow-up visits. At first, she brought her husband along with her to these sessions, but after a while she came alone. Later still, she appeared in the company of a young man.

When the follow-ups ended, I didn't see her in my office until more than a year after the operation. By that time, I'd discovered that she felt so sexy and attractive that she had left her husband and home to start a new life. She cultivated as many as three young boyfriends and eventually married one of them, some fifteen years her junior.

That new liaison did not last long. About ten years after I had first met her, she was divorced from her second husband. Her original family severed all ties with her; the last I heard of her, she was a miserable woman, an assistant in a Jerusalem department store.

The lesson I learned was that a successful plastic surgery operation can sometimes have unexpected (and certainly unintended) results that bring more harm than good.

VICTORY FROM DEFEAT

NARENDRA PANDYA, M.D. BOMBAY, INDIA

*We are generally the better persuaded by
the reasons to discover ourselves than
those given to us by others.*
–Pascal

One of the world's really tough jobs is laying ocean pipe. Long, eighteen-inch heavy steel pipes have to be maneuvered into position by floating crane, carefully aligned and bolted together, and finally lowered to the seabed. Not a task for wimps. The pipe layer has to have physical strength and endurance, an eye for perfect accuracy of alignment, and a sharp awareness of the dangers in working with heavy objects in an often unfriendly environment.

I was working in a Bombay hospital when I encountered one of these pipe layers, a man of about thirty-five, who had been flown in by helicopter after a serious accident. He had been working on a pipeline being constructed to bring oil from an offshore drill rig. A crane driver let slip one of the heavy pipe sections. This great metal cylinder fell on the one below, where the man was working. Both his hands were badly damaged, and all eight fingers were severed. Only his two thumbs remained.

As a surgeon, my first reaction was to find out whether it would be possible to retrieve the missing fingers, so that they would be available for reattaching. The operating managers were unanimous in their verdict that, no, that was quite out of the question. They were now lying, untraceable, on the bottom of the Indian Ocean.

Unable to pursue that line, I closed all the amputation stumps and had the man formally admitted as a patient into the hospital. As he recovered from surgery and the anesthetic wore off, I was immediately impressed by the quite extraordinary confidence and positive attitude he displayed, in spite of his devastating loss.

"Doctor," was his continuing refrain, "just do whatever you have to – I'm quite sure that I'll get back my job later." No self-pity, no moaning – just this quiet assurance that his demanding lifework would continue as it had before.

Clearly, then, my task was to achieve an optimum outcome from further surgery. I had many photographs taken of his injuries, which, supported by detailed information, I sent to many colleagues around the world, requesting their feedback. With this information from many expert perspectives, I carried out four operations in the next six months. I was satisfied that the best possible job had been done to help him overcome his disability.

When the time came for him to leave, I realized that he had reached a stage where he could use his hands postoperatively virtually as well as he could before the procedures. He left the hospital, went back to the same job, and now – ten years after the accident – he is still happy in his work.

The theme which underlies this story is not the accident, nor the surgery which followed. It is the strength and confidence of a man, who, in spite of such a debilitating injury, was never depressed, never despondent, nor did he blame the whole world for his misfortune.

In fact, he did not even feel that he had suffered a misfortune. He saw it as being just a roll of the dice and continued his life with the same courage and the same smile he had before.

My admiration for that man has never diminished.

FAIR COMPENSATION

ROBERT E. MALLIN, M.D.   SANTA FE, NM

A wise man sees as much as he ought,
not as much as he can.
–Montaigne

All plastic surgeons have experiences of great poignancy. For me, one of the most memorable of these was when a Filipino patient of mine brought his aunt back from her own country to see me in my office.

She was an extraordinary and pitiful sight to behold. At six years of age, she had been severely burned. Living in a remote village in the Philippines, she had received no treatment. Instead, her family had kept her isolated in a back room of their hut for almost fifty years – years in which her burn injuries had fossilized into permanent disability and disfigurement.

She had amazing contractures, of a type normally seen only in old-fashioned surgery textbooks, from her chin to her neck, her mouth to her chin, and all over her face. She was incapable of movement, she could hardly talk, and she salivated constantly.

Beyond these awesome physical factors, she was an unregistered/illegal immigrant into Alaska and had no insurance of any kind. Despite everything, we decided to try some surgery.

We had to sell the idea pretty hard, but the anesthesiologist agreed to do everything pro bono, as eventually did the hospital. We started on a long series of operations: her contractures were released, multiple graftings performed, dental work done.

The procedures were successful beyond our original hopes. She became able to speak and reached a point where she went shopping in the malls. In short, she was completely rehabilitated and had a good quality of life at age fifty-five, after all those years of imprisonment within her own body.

My proudest moment was when this re-born lady insisted on paying for the care we had given her by preparing the most magnificent feast of Filipino food that could be imagined. Helped by her relatives, she spread the delicacies all over the office, and we all enjoyed the exotic flavors of her native land.

THE RESPONSIBLE ADULT

ROBERT N. COOPER, M.D.   STUART, FL

*A man's worst difficulties begin when he is able
to do what he likes.*
–T. H. Huxley

Renee was the fifty-eight-year-old wife of a movie actor known for his tough-guy roles. In some respects, she replicated his gruff personality, but inside was a warm and mellow femininity. She came to me from her Miami home for a face-lift and eyelid rejuvenation, making a special point that she wanted to travel the hundred-mile journey south from my office as soon as she was out of sedation. Two friends were to collect her for the drive.

The procedure was uneventful. Although still somewhat sedated, Renee was quite coherent within thirty minutes of leaving the operating room. All the necessary dressings were in place; just two hours later, her two friends arrived as promised.

In the field of outpatient plastic surgery, it is accepted practice to discharge a patient only into the care of a "responsible adult" A mere taxi ride home would be unacceptable. I judged that the two ladies fell into the "responsible" category, and Renee was wheeled into the front passenger seat.

Off they went. But just forty-five minutes later, Renee reappeared at the office door – head dressing twisted, moistened eye sponges gone missing, and with a bruised forehead. What on earth had happened?

Before they had driven out of the parking lot, both "responsible adults" had signaled their lack of enthusiasm for the long drive. Renee's type A personality propelled her to take over the wheel, and – senses still rather askew from the effects of sedation – she drove off.

She soon realized that the car was low on fuel, and she pulled into a gas station before getting on the freeway. While circling the car to pay for the gas, she tripped on the hose and banged her head on the concrete pavement, sending her carefully applied dressings out of kilter. Nothing daunted, she dusted herself off and drove back to the office to see if any harm had been done. My patient coordinator and I were more than taken aback to see her again in this state – we were flabbergasted.

I examined her, found that there was no significant damage, adjusted and replaced the dressings, and finally got the lady to agree that she would either check into a local hotel or take the back seat in the car to Miami. Her warmth and rationality did battle with the type A factors and won. Miami it was – with her in a purely passenger role. When I saw her again two days later for a postoperative check, she, smiling, confided in me that she had found the whole episode quite amusing.

Inwardly, I was less than impressed. My definition of "responsible adult" had undergone a rapid revision.

FROZEN NORTH

ROBERT E. MALLIN, M.D.   SANTA FE, NM

Many are stubborn in pursuit of
the path they have chosen,
few in pursuit of the goal.
–Nietzsche

Tim, a Native American living in Fairbanks, Alaska, and a friend were driving on the road outside of town when their car caught fire. Both were severely burned.

The young men managed to get free of the burning vehicle, rolled in the snow to extinguish the flames, and, then, seeing that the car itself was not badly harmed, tried to get back inside to protect themselves from the freezing temperatures until help came along. But, to their horror, in their rush to smother their burning clothes in the snow they had locked themselves out. They walked for many miles, barefoot in the dead of winter, clothes burnt, skin damaged, until by good luck they were picked up by a passing trooper. They finally arrived at our hospital.

The driver's father happened to be a Medicaid executive. For reasons which are best not revealed here, the young man had all his treatment paid for. Tim, however, failed on some technicality to qualify for such financing. So all of the treatment team – consultants, burn unit, myself, everything – took care of him with no charge. The course of his recovery was difficult – on at least two occasions we resurrected him from "code 99s", the very edge of death. It was professionally dramatic and emotionally draining.

Tim was eventually restored to good health and left us to return to his reservation in South Dakota. I retired from practice and thought little more of the episode. However, after about eighteen months, Tim managed to trace my whereabouts and got in touch with me.

His first words were: "I think I owe you a bill."

I replied, "Oh, no, that was a long time ago. We treated you at no cost to you, as we knew that you had no insurance and no other way of paying."

But he persisted. At last, I interrupted him. "Look, this is ridiculous. Sure you owe nineteen thousand dollars, but I don't expect you to pay for it. Please accept your life with my compliments."

He would not let the matter drop. Invoking his native culture and spirits, he told me that he considered it a debt of honor to pay. I backed down, agreed to accept any payments that he could make, and told him that we would reduce the debt by two dollars for each dollar that he contributed – and that we would charge no interest on the outstanding debt.

Since that conversation, he has been paying fifty dollars at odd intervals over many years; and, as I write this story, he has brought the debt down to a few hundred dollars. The reward, however, has been much more than financial. Each year he sends me a family newsletter, with pictures. He works with drug-and-alcohol-addicted children. He is a swimming coach. He became Teacher of the Year at the reservation high school last year.

It is a rare and precious event in the life of any of us to be able to point to a life you saved and, through that outcome, to play a part in the creation of good things on this earth. For me, this was a true success story.

TRANSGENERATIONAL LOVE

STANLEY TAUB, M.D.   NEW YORK, NY

The man who lives free from folly, is not so wise as
he thinks.
    –La Rochefoucauld

A 58-year-old male rock musician came to me for a facelift.
His name was John P. Senior. He told me he was in a very
competitive, youth-oriented profession; in order to keep
working in the band, he had to disguise his age. This he did
with a long-haired wig and gigantic sideburns. However, his
older appearance was becoming more difficult to hide in
spite of his clever artifices.

I did a full facelift with eyelids; postoperatively, he looked
remarkably youthful. A few months later he came in for a
follow-up visit, bringing this beautiful 22-year-old girl with
him.

While she waited in the reception room, he took me aside
and told me that the young lady was his new wife and that
he had initially met her as John P. Senior a few months
before. During a gig he secretly fell in love with her. She of
course took him as a friendly, fatherly figure. He met her
again soon after the facelift. She didn't recognize him. He
told her he was John P. Senior's son, age 36, and that his
father, John P. Senior, had retired to California. They started dating, he proposed, and they got married. She had
hoped to see his father again at the wedding. Being a good
actor, he sadly told her that his father had passed away from
a sudden illness.

DIAGNOSIS BY GUN

SUSAN KOLB, M.D.   **ATLANTA, GA**

The difference between the mystical experience and the psychological crack-up is that the one who cracks is drowning in the water in which the mystic swims.
        —Joseph Campbell

One of my patients was a man who sustained an injury requiring the reimplantation of four fingers. As is often the case with accidents occurring at a place of employment, the patient was sent by the Worker's Compensation insurance company to their psychologist for an evaluation. This doctor decided that my patient had a problem with women, serious enough to need six to eight weeks of therapy.

To be frank, I could see no evidence that would support this conclusion. He had a normal, healthy relationship with his wife, and there was nothing out of context in his behavior with me – and we were the two most important women in his life at that point.

My patient decided to resolve the question in his own unusual way. After the psychologist had delivered his verdict, the injured man took a gun permit from his wallet and set it on the table. Then he slowly took out his gun and put it on the table as well, between himself and the psychologist.

The psychologist took a deep breath, told the patient that he had changed his mind, and that he now believed him to be completely normal psychologically and in no need of treatment.

A unique way of forcing a doctor to change his diagnosis without a word being spoken . . . .

INTUITION AND INSIGHT

SUSAN KOLB, M.D.   ATLANTA, GA

There is an often-quoted verse in sandscrit which appears in the Chinese Tao-te Ching as well: "He who thinks he knows, doesn't know. He who knows that he doesn't know, knows. For in this context, to know is not to know. And not to know is to know.
—Joseph Campbell

Some of our patients exhibit remarkable intuition and spiritual insight about their injuries, sources of knowledge which may be of a higher order than rational practicality. Let me tell you a story which illustrates what I mean.

I was called to the emergency room one day to help with a patient who had suffered a severe hand injury at work. When he reached the recovery phase, he told me that, on the morning of the accident, he had a powerful feeling that he should not go into work that day. Having a strong sense of responsibility, he disregarded the feeling, got into his car, but then just sat there, battling the intuition which would not go away.

He decided to follow his instinct and got out of the car – and immediately felt guilty, so he climbed back in. Out again, in again, until finally guilt and his sense of duty won the fight against intuition, and he drove to work.

Having arrived, he went into his building. The first thing that happened to him as he began his tasks for the day was that he suffered a very severe injury to his nondominant hand when it went through a laminating machine, de-gloving the entire hand, including his fingers.

My attendance at the emergency room was brought about because he was bleeding through the tourniquet which had been applied. The ER physicians were concerned because they were unable to control the bleeding; and, as a declared Jehovah's Witness, the patient would not accept a blood transfusion.

First thing I did when I arrived in the ER was to inject the three major nerves in the wrist with a Lidocaine-Marcaine combination. This allowed him to calm down, and, by relieving his pain, brought his blood pressure down as well. As a result, I was able to take off the tourniquet and to control the bleeding with simple pressure dressings.

We proceeded to surgery to repair multiple vascular and soft-tissue injuries, during which we struggled to restore the blood circulation to the thumb using multiple maneuvers, but without success. The thumb remained white, and no blood supply was visible through the microvascular repairs. The thumb, I should emphasize, was the worst part of his injury: The distal portion of the thumb was totally off the proximal phalanx, and the neurovascular bundles had been stretched tremendously.

In the recovery room, I explained to the patient that I didn't think we had managed to save his thumb, and I feared we might lose it, as I knew of nothing more that could be done.

Later, he told me that, at that time, he knew he wasn't going to lose his thumb. He did foresee, however, that he would lose one finger, but he didn't know which one. To our surprise, four days later the thumb gradually regained its blood supply and became pink and healthy-looking. At the same time, the ring finger gradually lost its circulation and began to necrose. Eventually, we had to amputate the ring finger at the level of the proximal phalanx.

I had been a hand surgeon for some seventeen years and a student of spiritual medicine for at least fifteen. Those years have given me the opportunity to study the spiritual significance of finger injuries.

References to these meanings are to be found in various esoteric texts, but instead of relying on them, I decided to test their hypothesis in real life. Spiritual medicine maintains that every injury has a spiritual significance, sometimes quite specific. Injuries of the thumb involve issues of will: of the index finger, faith; of the middle finger, self-love and worthiness; of the ring finger, physical and material security; and of the little finger, sexual and relationship issues.

In my many years as a hand surgeon, I've been able to observe and work with many patients who sustained finger injuries. Often I've found that the spiritual lesson of each finger has a great deal of meaning to the patient.

Returning to the case of my patient who had the argument with a laminating machine, I learned that he was dealing with physical and material security issues in his life, not so much with issues of will. On the morning of his injury, he had not paid attention to the intuition warning him to stay home. Therefore the thumb, although damaged, was not lost. Since then, I have treated many patients who have told me similar stories about instinctive warning signals which, if they had not ignored them, would have saved them from sustaining accident injuries.

I believe that all of us – especially surgeons – should pay

attention to the intuition which is given to us before, say, a particularly delicate or dangerous procedure, telling us that we should not use the knife. So many times we say to ourselves, "I knew I should not have done that."

The spiritual lesson taught on these occasions is that we should develop our sense of the intuitive, which ultimately will protect us even in those circumstances where our intellect cannot.

THE SPIRITUAL DIMENSION

SUSAN KOLB, M.D.   ATLANTA, GA

More than in any time in history, mankind faces a crossroad. One path heads to despair and utter hopelessness, the other to total extinction. Let us pray that we have the wisdom to choose correctly.
–Woody Allen

The female patient who came to me desiring a breast augmentation was unusual in one major respect. She had recently been released from prison, where she had served a term for financial fraud.

She was very straightforward in recounting this part of her history to me and told me that, after five years in prison, she wanted to do something nice for herself. Hence her request for breast augmentation.

I examined her and found that she was a good candidate for this procedure. She asked me to use an axillary approach, as she did not want any scars on her breasts. We agreed on a transaxillary submuscular augmentation, using silicone gel implants. We arranged that the operation would take place the next day, and then we said our farewells.

It was my habit to meditate before going to bed. That night, during my meditation, I was shown that she would have a complication on her right breast. With my mind's eye, I saw a capsular contracture form – a common enough difficulty, but one about which I had never previously been forewarned before the operation.

120

Still in meditative mode, I asked if I should do the operation in view of the advance knowledge that there would be a complication. A response came:

"Yes, she has to learn to detach from the physical."

The following day, the operation was carried out with no problem, and my patient did well for a week. Then her uncle pulled her arm with some force, which led to a swelling on the right side. A little later, this developed into a mild but noticeable capsular contracture.

Needless to say, she was not happy at the asymmetry caused by the contracture and asked if I could fix the problem. This was in the days before the endoscope was widely used, so I told her that I could, but that the procedure would leave a scar on the lower part of the breast.

This gave her a dilemma with a spiritual dimension: a choice of living with the capsular contracture, or having a scar on her breast in an area which she felt would be visible. Either way, she would "detach from the physical."

This experience brought me to the realization that we are often put in such situations when it is time for us to learn our spiritual lessons. We will learn them, whatever choice we make.

As plastic surgeons, we cannot always prevent our patients' complications even if we know about them in advance. However, if we are aware that such lessons are taking place, we can help our patients through them. I believe that plastic surgery is a specialty which is unique in giving opportunities to help not only with people's physical needs, but with their emotional, mental, and, yes, spiritual challenges as well.

THE MAN WITH NO FACE

WILLIAM J. HOSTNIK, M.D.
NEW LONDON, CT

*Everybody is perfectly willing to learn from unpleas-
ant experiences – if only the damage of the first lesson could be repaired.*
  –Lichtenberg

Alcohol and lawn mowing do not go so well together.
Certainly not in the case of Gus, a patient of mine who presented himself with an injury unique in my expenence.

Gus was an affable, good-natured, sixty-year-old black man
who had imbibed a little more than was good for him just
before setting to work cutting the grass on a hillside. No
sooner had he started the job than he slipped and fell. The
big mowing machine fell right on his face, blades whirring.

One doesn't need much imagination to picture the damage.
He was quickly brought into the emergency room of the
small-town hospital nearby.

I saw him in the ER. Little of his face and forehead were left.
The nose was gone; facial skin was badly chewed up and
lying off to one side, beside the left ear; a sizable part of the
forehead had been sliced off, together with at least half of
the frontal lobes of his brain. The exposed brain tissues were
full of grass clippings and clumps of dirt. Surprisingly, both
eyes and eyelids were in place.

In effect, Gus had undergone an informal prefrontal loboto-
my. When I saw him, he was fully conscious and uncon-

cerned with his plight. He was alert, and talking with complete clarity. Whether his reaction was caused by the damage to his brain, or was simply his normal sunny nature shining through, was hard to tell. Whatever the reason, it was highly unusual to come across a patient with such severe injuries taking so optimistic a view of his situation.

The immediate challenge, obviously, was to cover the brain.

Gus was anesthetized and cleansed in the operating room. The neurosurgeon covered the bone with a specially formulated plastic. I then moved a portion of the scalp to cover the open wound. I found that the skin which had been displaced to the front of the left ear had enough subcutaneous tissue to close the rest of the forehead. With some of the remaining skin, we were able to close the cheek areas.

We dealt with the missing nose by using what was left of the tissues to cover the gaps, allowing for future reconstruction. That left the upper lip, which was gone completely, but we postponed repair so as not to overstress the patient on this initial procedure – which he tolerated very well.

In subsequent operations, I was able to move the scalp back into its normal position and put a skin graft on the area so that he didn't have his scalp way down to just above the eyebrow. Then, months later, I used a cross-lip flap of tissue to repair the upper lip, using a turned-up portion of the lower lip, which had escaped injury.

Final reconstruction was to do something about the nose. I used a method known as a Tagliacozzi procedure - which I had never done before – and I believe that very few of us ever have. It involved using a part of his left arm to fashion a "new" nose; after defatting procedures and a strip of bone graft several months later, it turned out to be very satisfactory.

During all five months of this process, Gus had no problem handling the various operations. Were we seeing a new and pleasantly lobotomized personality? Or was it his naturally placid and friendly character?

It was unfortunate that a year later he suffered a stroke and died. But I shall always remember him, remember his dramatic disfigurement and brain . . . and in my mind's eye, see him smiling through it all!

SENSITIVITY TRAINING

MARJORIE CRAMER, M.D.   BROOKLYN, NY

Tact consists of knowing how far
to go in going too far.
—Cocteau

I was pregnant with both of my daughters during residency, one on General Surgery and one on Plastics. When I went to tell Dr. Bromberg about the second pregnancy, I assumed that my track record would stand me in good stead. I had worked at least as hard as the other residents throughout the first pregnancy and had taken only my 2 weeks vacation off for the delivery.

Imagine my surprise when he exclaimed that it was not enough that he had to teach his residents plastic surgery, but that he also had to teach them about birth control. My second daughter, now a 26-year-old psychologist, particularly enjoys this story. Once, after a very long and tedious procedure, the patient told me that it was comforting for him to feel my fetus moving though my large abdomen, which must have been leaning against his arm.

HIDDEN AGENDA

JOEL H. PAULL, M.D.   BUFFALO, NY

We wholly conquer only what we assimilate.
–Gide

About five years into my plastic surgical practice, I was approached by a registered nurse who sought consultation with regards to a facelift and eyelid rejuvenation. She seemed quite knowledgeable, although I had never had the opportunity of working with her in a hospital setting. She had no qualms about understanding the limitations as I pointed them out, or the potential complications. As a matter of interest, the only requirement that she insisted upon was that the surgery take place on the specified date. Although I could not understand her needs in that regard, I saw no reason not to comply and scheduled her accordingly.

The procedure took place as scheduled and went very smoothly. In the postoperative period she did very well and there were no problems at all. Drains and sutures came out at appropriate intervals and the result was very pleasing. The patient returned to my office for follow-up visits and expressed her delight with her appearance.

After one month of follow-up I had asked her to return again in approximately four to six weeks for an additional follow-up visit and was astounded when she entered the office complaining bitterly that she had gone through all of this surgery and felt that nothing had been achieved. She accused me of performing inadequate surgery and suggested that I should be ashamed of myself for taking the fee for little or no results. Her unabated bitterness was obvious to me. She would not have a reasonable discussion and continually berated the results of her surgery, which on her previous visit had been praised to the skies.

This seemingly logical, intelligent and erstwhile sophisticated patient was now the bane of my existence. She threatened a lawsuit and only after careful reflection of the fact that I was really quite pleased with the results achieved and saw no evidence whatsoever of any untoward result, did I resist her statements and, although I offered to continue to care for her, I did tell her that if she could not behave in a more appropriate fashion, it would be necessary to sever our doctor patient relationship.

Nothing more was heard from the patient, but approximately six months later, in a very unplanned fashion, another nurse sought my consultation and relayed that she had seen my earlier patient and was quite impressed with the result. I silently listened as she suggested that I might enjoy being aware of the fact that my patient, too, had now come about to being pleased with the result. I said that was very nice but I had not seen my patient is several months. It was then explained to me, unbeknownst to my new patient what light she was shedding on my confusion, that my earlier patient had been seeing a married man prior to her surgery with me. On the specific day she insisted her surgery be performed, her paramour had left on an extended 30 day vacation with his wife. When he returned, he did not, as my patient expected, drop his wife and run off with my patient, but instead the relationship broke off.

This was the most intimate experience I had come to understand as to the unspoken objective that a patient may never discuss with the surgeon.Henceforward, and for many years, I always took the care to explain to prospective surgical patients that not only could we not guarantee the results, but we certainly cannot achieve objectives with which we are not familiar. The lesson has served me very well and it might well perhaps be something that others may wish to think about.

TOP GUN, TOP THUMB

HARRY J. BUNCKE, M.D.   SAN MATEO, CA

HARRY J. BUNCKE, M.D.   SAN MATEO, CA

It is best for great men to shoot over,
and for lesser men to shoot short.
–Halifax

I would like to illustrate how a toe-to-thumb transplant can change a person's life. This story concerns a Lieutenant Colonel in the Navy Air Force. He was a fighter pilot flying F14s in the Vietnamese War and was an outstanding pilot. As a matter of fact, he did the flying of the F14s in the movie Top Gun. Hoser Cetroppa, as he was called, was also an avid hunter. He liked to build his own dens and he liked to hunt with bows and arrows and rifles. He hunted deer, elk, and bear. He was building himself a new type of rifle with a slide lock on it and, unfortunately, the first time he fired it the bolt blew loose, fired off posteriorly, and tore off his thumb at the metacarpal phalangeal joint level, and destroyed the whole proximal portion of his index finger.

The Navy sent him to us for an acute injury. Unfortunately, we could not replant anything, but we were able to use the destroyed index finger to fillet it and cover the missing dorsum of the hand, for he had multiple metacarpal fractures, but here he is with his missing thumb and only three fingers left on his hand. Well, I don't know if you know any fighter pilots but they are a high energy group of people. Flying was Hoser's life and there he was with his dominant hand blown up. He was contemplating suicide. Well, after a few months, when he settled down, we actually went to the naval hospital in Oakland and performed a large toe transplant, taking the first metatarsal joint because he had blown away his

129

metacarpal bone, and giving him a long thumb.

This gentleman was so dedicated that he went back and re-qualified as a fighter pilot down in Pensacola, going through the whole training again, and was all set to go to the Gulf War when it ended. Of course, he was happy the war was over, but he couldn't wait to get back into his F18. We actually went to Fallon, which is a Navy Air Force base out in the deserts of Nevada, hundreds of miles from anywhere, and he showed us some of the flight training exercises they have there, which are really astounding. Incidentally, while he was waiting to have his operation, the press got word of it and Connie Chung, who is a reporter of international note, went to the Naval hospital in Oakland to interview Hoser. She said to him, "Well, Mr. Cetroppa, suppose the operation is a failure and you lose your toe. Now you're missing a toe and a thumb." Hoser's comment, without blinking an eye, was "Well I've got another big toe. We'll go for that one." He is that kind of guy. He is really an inspiration.

Of course, he was retired from the Naval Air Force after the Gulf War and he joined the Forest Service flying Borag Bombers. He has been doing that for, oh, ten years or more, and he says it is almost as much fun as flying fighter jets. He dives into these valleys and bombs forest fires with water.

He is living life his way. I don't know what he's going to do when he retires, provided he lives till retirement. Every year the Forest Service loses one or two Borag Bombers. Recently, Hoser was flying out of a ravine when he hit a pine tree, chopping off about ten feet of his wing. It was a given that he was able to fly the plane safely back to base. Mentally, he is beyond a doubt one of the toughest men I have ever encountered.

DOROTHY

THOMAS J. KRIZEK, M.D. TAMPA, FL

Beholding beauty with the eye of the mind . . .
  –Plato

In May of 1976, Mrs. Dorothy S., a 69-year-old married housewife, underwent an upper and lower lid blepharoplasty (eyelid lift). She was extraordinarily pleased with herself and with the operation. On reflection, I feel it was the finest operation that I performed in the forty-three years in which I have been involved in surgery. The residents awarded me the "Golden Hand" award for the single most memorable procedure that they had witnessed that year at Yale. Let me share the rest of the story with you.

In any career in plastic surgery, there are, not surprisingly, a handful of patients that shape the course of that career. Dorothy, Susan, Hans and Helen, Norb, K-29 and Frank were all memorable to me. These people (all humans except K-29, a dog) shaped mine.

In sequence, Susan was my longest effort at craniofacial reconstruction BEFORE Tessier, the Parisian "father" of craniofacial surgery. Hans and Helen were exposed to 250,000 rads of radiation therapy. On Norb, I performed a skin flap and used it to carry muscle. It was a myocutaneous (skin and muscle) flap, which I named incorrectly, and thus missed the opportunity for discovery. On the mongrel dog K-29, my teacher, Clifford Kiehn, and I performed the first microvascular free flap. And Frank was a successful reconstruction of an Andy Gump deformity (Andy was a cartoon character with no chin).

Each of these patients taught me something special about my art that only he or she could teach me. But most special of them all was Dorothy.

Dorothy came to me shortly after my arrival at Yale as Chief of Plastic Surgery in the late 1960s. She had previously undergone removal of part of her jaw and floor of the mouth, with a radical neck dissection of lymph nodes, followed by radiation. She had been free of disease for a couple of years and she wanted reconstruction of the jaw. I thought her to be a suitable candidate.

I determined that she was deficient of tissue, both internal lining and soft tissue coverage, and I set about to correct this with a series of regional flaps to be followed by bone grafting.

Dorothy and I did not face the limitations of managed care and "length of stay"; Dorothy's stays were often long-term. Her relationship with the nurses, staff and residents on the second floor of the Tompkins building of the Yale-New Haven Hospital became close and warm. Dorothy's husband, like she before her cancer, drank heavily (which increases the risk of mouth cancer) and was often absent for long periods.

In fact, her home life lacked intimacy and support. Friends drifted away as Dorothy's deformity and difficulty in talking made close contact uncomfortable for them. Dorothy found herself less and less willing to go about daily tasks. She began to avoid the pain of meeting people in stores, in church, and on the street, who recoiled when they recognized that she was disfigured. It began to seem like only those of us on Tompkins-2 recognized Dorothy by her name and as one of us. Over time, we all forgot that Dorothy looked different. Dorothy, like so many disfigured and deformed, recognized her difference reluctantly and was unaware of it much of the time, as long as others did not affirm it.

Dorothy's operations were largely unsuccessful. Bone grafts eroded through the newly placed flaps; although flaps were viable, they were not able to support the new blood supply to the bone. I attempted to design and transfer a flap that contained a portion of the collarbone as a composite flap. It failed. I designed a tubed pedicle flap from skin on her abdomen, transferred it to the wrist as a carrier, and then watched in sorrow as the entire flap died on the abdomen following the final delay.

Dorothy was too early for microvascular free transfer — the technique of separating a portion of the body and "plugging in" the arteries, veins and nerves to cover another area with a defect. Although I had performed it on a dog, I failed to recognize until much later the potential for humans.

She was also too early for myocutaneous flap transfer. Although I had performed one on Norb's thigh, I had thought that the skin was used to carry the muscle instead of the other way around. I alone was responsible for the failures, which occurred in spite of the able assistance of Robson, Ariyan, Koss, Frazier, Edstrom, McGrath and Walton, all of whom to this day will smile when I say "Dorothy," since they too shared the many years' experience of knowing her.

For Dorothy became a friend to us. She demonstrated an incredible fortitude that enabled her to continue on when society was unable to accept her deformity, and when my surgery was unable to relieve her disfigurement. She demonstrated a human dignity few of us had seen before in others, and she made a continued demand, believing that it is the divine right of humans to look normal. And that is, of course, what our specialty has been all about.

It was many years into her ongoing efforts at jaw reconstruction that Dorothy asked me to correct her baggy eyelids. She taught me that by looking past her other disfigurement, I would see a vibrant, determined woman who cared about her appearance. Why, indeed, should she not also benefit from aesthetic surgery?

Dorothy's story eventually came to an end. Early in 1978 I made plans to move to Columbia-Presbyterian Medical Center in New York, and offered Dorothy the opportunity to continue her care there. It was only a short distance farther from her home than her trip to New Haven. She considered the alternative of remaining at Yale with the many friends she had made, to be cared for by colleagues who knew her as well as I. Dorothy felt that neither choice was agreeable, and become very sad about the changes that were to occur.

Unexpectedly, ten years after our almost simultaneous arrival at Yale, she developed a recurrence of her cancer and died. Dorothy bracketed my decade at Yale and punctuated my departure. I remember Yale more than fondly. I'd had the privilege of working with the residents and medical students, the incredible nurses, physicians' assistants and other colleagues. There was the experience of being part of a great University.

But the dearest of all these was Dorothy. She taught us to look beyond an obvious defect and see something more subtle.

Chapter IV

Chance

A PROFOUND ABLUTION

ABDEL RAOUF ISMAIL, M.D.
DHAHRAN, SAUDI ARABIA

The greatest difficulties lie where we
are not looking for them.
–Goethe

A young male was brought to our Dhahran emergency room with burns to the genitalia and the buttocks region, together with spotty involvement of the thighs. Initially, the nature of the burns was not clear, but after a while the patient offered an illuminating history.

He explained that when he was about to wash his genitalia in preparation for the Moslem prayer, he reached out for a pot of water and started the cleansing ritual. Unfortunately for him, the water-pot had been replaced by another container, full of a chemical whose nature was unknown to the patient.

It later transpired that the plumbing in his house had developed an obstruction, and plumbers had been called in to fix the problem. The plumbers had used a powerful alkali, contained in a pot the same size and color as the waterpot. When they left, the workmen had mistakenly taken the water and left the chemical. The result was that the young man had poured strong alkali over his genitals.

Initial treatment of the injuries was conservative, but eventually he required skin grafting of the glans penis, the shaft, and spots over his thighs and scrotum.

Custom dictates that Moslems wash their face, ears, neck, hands, feet and genitalia five times daily before prayers. In the Arabic tongue, this is known as "wuzu," or ablution, in preparation for prayer. In following the rites of his religion, this poor fellow had done serious damage to his genital area.

Ablution may be a good thing, but a deep chemical burn – especially in such a sensitive area – is too much.

ALIEN M.D.

EDMOND A. ZINGARO, M.D.
SAN FRANCISCO, CA

A prudent man will think more important what
fate has conceded to him than what it has denied.
–Gracian

Back in the late eighties, I was still taking plastic surgery emergency room calls. One night, I was paged to see a young man who had been in an automobile accident and sustained severe facial injuries.

Apparently this sixteen year old had been driving in the wintry, snowy mountains. He'd been driving carefully and slowly enough, but he hit black ice while making a turn. The car slid out of control and fell over on its side. The glass broke; he was dragged, face exposed to the unforgiving road surface, until the vehicle hit an embankment and stopped.

When I arrived at the facility where he'd been taken, I saw a sight that was quite literally out of *Alien*. The boy's face was torn to pieces. It was so badly damaged that all the soft tissues had been peeled away from around one eye, and that eye was circumferentially exposed.

He was stabilized and then taken to surgery, where I joined a number of other different specialists. We worked for hours trying to put everything back together.

He was in the hospital a long time and underwent several further surgical procedures before being discharged home.

That was not the end of it, however. Over the next year or so, I performed several more reconstructive operations on him. Then time went by, I moved to San Francisco, and we lost track of one another.

Years later found me in another hospital, checking on a patient. A young man with long red hair tied in a ponytail, and wearing the white coat of a resident, came up to me. He spoke.

"Dr Zingaro, do you remember me?"

His face rang a bell from the distant past. I thought I recognized him in spite of the modest but evident facial deformities, but I almost fell over when I read the name on his ID badge. It was the car accident man!

The accident and its aftermath had not prevented him from completing college and medical school – he was now a resident in psychiatry. He went on to thank me for all the work I'd done and told me how pleased he was with the way everything had turned out.

It was a particularly touching moment when he said that meeting me and going through the traumatic processes of facial surgery had helped him decide to go into medicine. He shared the story with his fellow residents in training, as well as with his attending staff physicians. While they were all affected by what he had to say, what I was feeling inside was overwhelming.

I now bump into my former patient turned colleague quite regularly. Each time, I cannot avoid thinking that this young doctor is the very epitome of a success story.

A TALE OF TWO CITIES

ROGER SIMPSON, M.D.   GARDEN CITY, NY

> *One real world is enough.*
> –Santayana

"All animals are equal, but some are more equal than others." *In Animal Farm*, George Orwell sums up the human condition with a degree of cynicism. The inequalities of the world are sometimes brought home to the plastic surgeon in a starkly dramatic way.

Peter and Rafael live in two cities – the first world and the third. Rafael's Santo Domingo is the capital of the Dominican Republic, sharing the island of Hispaniola with dirt-poor and misgoverned Haiti. The Dominican Republic's growing prosperity is markedly skewed; like so many third world countries, the rich get richer, the poor, poorer. At least a quarter of Dominicans eke out a miserable existence below the poverty line. Peter, in vivid contrast, lives in the United States.

Some time back, I got a telephone call from a high school girl who was doing missionary work in Santo Domingo. She was devoting her summer to a church facility which cared for "discarded" children. During her service, she encountered Rafael, a young man of nineteen who, a year previously, had been burned in a house fire caused by an explosion in the primitive oven.

Rafael had no education, no opportunity. Even without his

injuries, the outlook for his future would have been bleak. Medical care for him consisted of nothing beyond being looked after by his siblings. He lived, after all, in the poorest of the poor parts of his country. Even though his burns had only affected twenty percent of his body, less than catastrophic in medical treatment terms, he was not expected to live. Both arms and hands had been burned, as well as small areas of his face. His brothers and sisters took time off from school to feed him and to change his dressings.

It was, of course, not enough. Six months after the accident, most of the burn areas had superficially repaired themselves. But he had developed such severe scars that he could not bring his hand to his mouth. Even if he could have performed this simple act, his thumb could not touch his fingers on either hand.

The high school girl's intervention gave him a second chance. Through the church, the local diocese, and the Dominican community in our area we were able to make arrangements to bring him to the United States, where he would have the hope of rebuilding his damaged limbs and face . . . and his life.

The day he arrived, I had a therapist make a device that enabled him to feed himself for the first time in a year. At that early stage in his rehabilitation, my staff and I felt a wave of deep emotion as he tried to thank us for such a simple act. That emotion was compounded when we realized that his greatest relief was that he would be able to release his small brother from the role of caregiver and get him back to school.

Our continuing surgical efforts for Rafael over a long period of time have met with great successes, but an almost equal number of setbacks. Even with the asset of youth, the disfiguring scars and the contracted fragile joints do not easily return to normal. But throughout the treatment, he has always been smiling, always optimistic.

Now let us step back into the first world. The reason the school girl contacted me in the first place was that, several years earlier, I had taken care of her twelve-year-old brother Peter. Peter had sustained seventy percent burns while fooling around with gasoline. He not only survived; he flourished.

Although he had to undergo many reconstructive procedures, he called upon his reserves of intelligence and opportunity, graduated from Amherst and went on to Berkeley. As he matured through the teenage years and into manhood, he used his inevitable deformities to his advantage and chose to postpone the completion of reconstructive surgery until he finished college.

If Rafael had been born into Peter's situation and suffered his relatively minor burns (twenty versus seventy percent) in a more privileged community, his wounds would have been excised after two days and immediately grafted with new skin. Within two weeks, chances are that most of the grafts would have healed well. A program of therapy would have ensured that after a few months he would have been functioning at a high level.

The accident of birth into poverty in a country with limited resources was the key difference between the outcomes of Rafael and Peter. Rafael will ultimately become more functional and achieve a limited degree of normal life. Peter is already living it.

These two episodes burned two emotions into the minds of all of those – myself included – involved in the care of Rafael. One is a reaffirmation of the life-enhancing power of plastic surgery, even when it has to overcome the late start of the boy from Santo Domingo. The other is the chasm that exists in medical care between the first and third worlds.

A tale of two cities, indeed. But more than that, it is a parable of the way change, the roll of the human dice, inflicts injustice.

GRATITUDE

JANA K. RASMUSSEN, M.D.
WEST PALM BEACH, FL

I went to a general surgery residency program that was a Yale affiliate. It was a nice community hospital and we had several rotations through Yale, one being plastic surgery for three months in our second year of general surgery. At this time, I studied under Dr. Stephan Ariyan and at that time his chief resident, Zana Chicarelli. Like most plastic surgeons at that time, I was extremely compulsive, very organized, and pretty much of a perfectionist in everything I did.

I'd like to think it was the fact that I was a great resident that I was noticed by Dr. Ariyan, but I think it was my attention to detail and sense of organizational skills that actually made me an effective resident. Anyway, during my fourth year of general surgery residency, when one has to think about what they are going to do in their future, Dr. Ariyan approached me while I was doing a cardiac surgery rotation at Yale. He asked if I would be interested in one of the positions in the plastic surgery residency program after I completed my general surgery residency. I told him I would think about it. Of course, my first week of thinking, I was so honored by this offer that I was going to say yes. During the second week, I thought, "Wait a minute. I've never wanted to be a plastic surgeon." During the third week, I went back and forth on a see-saw and couldn't make up my mind.

144

I went to him at week four and had a rather lengthy conversation about my thoughts. I told him that I believed he should select someone who had wanted to be a plastic surgeon all their lives because they would probably be a better plastic surgeon. He did not agree. I also told him that, after all the training (in particular, five years of general surgery), that I didn't know if I wanted to pursue any further training programs, as it certainly impacted my personal life, at which point he stated that the profession of plastic surgery was an extremely great surgical specialty in that it could be tailored to fit anyone's personal needs. One could go into academic medicine, one could go into areas of plastic surgery which were less demanding, it would be easier to take sabbaticals.

He gave multiple reasons why plastic surgery was much better than any number of surgical specialties or general surgery.

I also had a relative lack of self-confidence and didn't know if I could successfully complete a plastic surgery program. Dr. Ariyan was very supportive and said that I had all the necessary criteria to be a skilled plastic surgeon. After about an hour of talking with him in his office, he convinced me that I should accept the position, which I did. His last comments to me during that meeting were, "Someday, you'll thank me."

This all took place in approximately 1984, and I started my plastic surgery residency in 1985, completing it in 1987. I moved from cold Connecticut to sunny south Florida, initially worked in a multi-specialty group as their sole plastic surgeon for three years, and then went out on my own in solo practice. Indeed, I found that I could easily organize my schedule so that I had very few emergencies, except, of course, when I had to cover the emergency room. I saw my

colleagues in general surgery or the other specialties working extremely hard, but not appearing to be extremely
happy. I, on the other hand, had a comfortable practice that
integrated with my personal life and I enjoyed what I did —
a very novel concept in this day and age of medicine when
many physicians have lost their zest for practicing medicine.

Several years later (in September, 1993), at the Annual
ASPRS Conference in New Orleans, I attended the reception
at The Aquarium. Far across the room, I saw Dr. Stephan
Ariyan, whom I hadn't seen since having completed my plastic surgery residency. I made my way through the crowd.
He was talking with another individual, but I stepped up to
him and he turned to me and said, "You're welcome."

Indeed, I am very thankful for him talking me into going to
plastic surgery. What other profession is so diverse, so rewarding, that we can make such a difference in our patients' lives?

CHANCE LED ME TO PLASTIC SURGERY

SIR WILLIAM MANCHESTER, KBE
AUCKLAND, NEW ZEALAND

He that leaveth nothing to chance will do few
things ill, but he will do very few things.
–Halifax

Until the Second World War, plastic surgical services in New Zealand were almost nonexistent and provided only in the private sector. My only knowledge of plastic surgery was that a New Zealander, Sir Harold Gillies, was famous in plastic surgery in London.

Now comes the story of how I did not choose plastic surgery, but how plastic surgery chose me. I had joined the New Zealand Medical Corps in February 1940 and was posted to a field ambulance at Burnham Military Camp near Christchurch. I was to leave in the Second Echelon, but circumstances relegated me to the Third Echelon, leaving at the end of 1940. Then comes the first in a chain of events which, though I did not know it at the time, was to set the pattern for the rest of my life.

The medical officer of the 22nd Battalion became drunk one Saturday night, not for the first time. The commanding officer was a fire-eater and a strict disciplinarian. When he saw this man unconscious and still in a drunken stupor when he was supposed to take the 6:00 A.M. sick parade the following morning, he exploded and demanded his replacement. I took his place. In this way, I was restored to the Second

Echelon, sailing in May 1940 in a large convoy for Egypt.

We sailed across the Tasman Sea. Off Sydney, our already large convoy of ships (*Aquitania, Empress of Britain, Empress of Japan*, and *Andes*) was joined by the *Queen Mary, Mauretania,* and *Empress of Canada*, full of Australian troops also sailing to Egypt. After rounding the southwest corner of Australia, we entered the Indian Ocean.

At about the time we reached the Cocos Islands, France fell and the Dunkirk evacuation was about to take place. The authorities decided that the Australian and New Zealander troops already on the water were much more urgently needed in the United Kingdom, so we were diverted around the Cape of Good Hope to provide a mobile reserve in case of invasion by Hitler. This was the second in the chain of events.

The Director of Medical Services in the Second Echelon was John Twhigg, a classmate of Archie McIndoe, who was himself a relative and partner of Sir Harold Gillies. Naturally, on arrival John Twhigg visited his classmate where he learned that surgeons from Australia, Canada, and South Africa were already being trained under the overall supervision of Sir Harold Gillies. When John Twhigg asked what sort of a New Zealander surgeon should be sent, he replied, "I want a promising, practical, commonsense young surgeon without much experience in general surgery, and then I won't have the impossible task of unteaching him all his bad habits." They looked around for such a person, but couldn't find one. In desperation they chose me.

When this proposition was put to me I was inclined to reject it and asked for a week to consider it. I decided to accept and, towards the end of 1940, found myself training in the plastic surgical unit at East Grinstead under Archie McIndoe, consultant to the R.A.F. After six months training helping to look after burned pilots, I was transferred to St. Albans under Mr. Rainsford Mowlem, another New Zealander. This was the second of three plastic surgery units around the periphery of London. A number of dental surgeons were being trained there, and Geoff Gilbert was amongst them.

Towards the end of 1941, Gilbert and I were asked to set up a plastic surgery unit in Helwan, Egypt, where we treated burns, facial fractures, and extensive soft-tissue injuries associated with compound fractures.

On the 23rd of October 1942 Field Marshall Montgomery and the Eighth Army opened the assault on EI Alamein, which led to the Germans being driven out of Africa. This was really the turning point of the whole war and we began to win from that moment onward.

I remained in Egypt for two years before being recalled to New Zealand to become second in command of a military plastic unit at Burwood near Christchurch. Towards the end of 1944 I was elevated to the rank of Lt. Colonel in command of this 30-bed unit. In 1946 I was discharged from the army and given the task of organizing the first properly constituted civilian plastic unit in the New Zealand Hospital service, expanding it from 30 to 60 beds. This had the effect of bringing plastic surgery services to ordinary New Zealanders in the same way as the existing specialities in the public hospital system. In 1947 the Unit had a visit from Field Marshall Lord Montgomery of Alamein.

At the end of 1947, I left Burwood to take up postgraduate

study in the United Kingdom, including a year at my old alma mater at East Grinstead. While there, early in 1950, the Auckland Hospital Board advertised the post of part-time stipendiary plastic surgeon at Middlemore Hospital in Auckland. It required the applicant to spend six-tenths of his time there. I applied and, about the middle of 1950, I received this letter from the Auckland Hospital Board dated the 21st June 1950. It reads as follows:

"I have much pleasure in confirming my cable of the 20th advising that you have been appointed to the position of Part-time Stipendiary Plastic Surgeon, Middlemore Hospital, from the 30th November 1950. You will be remunerated at the rate of one thousand pounds per annum."

I was thus able to take up my appointment almost exactly ten years after I first started at East Grinstead in 1940 during the Battle of Britain, well after half a century ago.

I spent the next twenty-eight years developing the unit, first to thirty beds and then to sixty and making a specialty of cleft lip and palate surgery. It was all very rewarding.

Thus, I was given a life in plastic surgery by that medical officer's drunkenness in Trentham Camp in 1940. Without his sacking, none of this would have happened.

There will always be a special place in my heart for that man!

Chapter V

Physician as Doctor – Doing One's Job

TRUNK CALL

HOLLIS H. CAFFEE, M.D.
GAINESVILLE, FL

Nature's great masterpiece, an elephant,
the only harmless great thing.
—John Donne

When I was first swept into this adventure, my mind dredged up from childhood memories a couplet which had much amused me all those years back:

Ellie the elephant's packed her trunk,
She's going to join the <u>cir</u> - cus...

We children would recite it with heavy emphasis on the first syllable of "circus," which impressed us as lending reality to the concept.

It was a fine morning in the summer of 1998 when I had a telephone call from the surgeons at the School of Veterinary Medicine.

"Doctor Caffee, this is going to sound like a very strange request."

The caller hesitated. I waited; there was silence on the line. Then he went on: "We have an elephant which has sustained an accidental amputation of the end of its trunk. We'd like your help in performing a reimplantation."

Again, silence. My first reaction was that this was some sort of practical joke.

"You can't be serious, can you? I mean, if you're wasting my time with some sort of hoax, I'm not going to be very happy − I've a busy practice here, you know."

"Hey, Doctor, we're serious all right. It may sound way out to you, but for the elephant patient it's a matter of life and death. She feeds herself by grasping food with the end of her trunk acting very much like a hand. Unless we can reconstruct the trunk, this lady will starve to death − hand-feeding is not a long-term option...will you help?"

This convinced me that the situation was real and urgent. I had a momentary vision of the animal lumbering into casualty, with myself seated on her as some sort of medical mahout, so we quickly agreed that the best thing was for me to bring some equipment to the patient and assess the best action we could take.

I was driven to the practice zoo, which was the elephant's home. The veterinary surgeon in charge told me that the accident had occurred some time during the previous night, although there was uncertainty about exactly when. Only by mid-morning did someone think to put the amputated part in the refrigerator.

I inspected the amputated part and the elephant herself − a gentle giantess! − and then examined the trunks of uninjured elephants. Clearly re-implantation would be technically feasible, as the arterial and venous systems were capable of reconnection.

But − and it was a big "but" − the trunk's nerves are large, and the nervous control of its intrinsic muscles highly complex. The muscles are capable of moving in all sorts of directions, and so the nerves have to be able to respond to sensation and translate these responses into exquisitely controlled movements. To give an example: An elephant can pick up a peanut, crack it, and remove the nut from the shell using only the end of its trunk, a maneuver difficult to achieve with the human hand.

For all of these reasons, we decided that reimplantation would not be in the elephant's best interests.

Our patient's damaged trunk looked like a double-barreled shotgun. An uninjured trunk, however, has a tip with the appearance of lips, with quite stiff edges. So we decided to go ahead with an operation to reshape the stump to restore it to a more normal appearance – and, hopefully, to a good degree of functionality.

Just like a surgical procedure on a human patient, general anesthesia first had to be induced. This was, without a doubt, the most fascinating part of this entire project. The veterinary anesthetist used a drug he referred to as M-99. A relatively small syringe demonstrated the awesome potency of this drug, since within seconds the animal was ready to drop.

The staff had anticipated this, and had a crew in the pen with a large wooden pallet. They were able to make sure that the elephant landed on the pallet and not on the ground, which allowed them to pick her up with a forklift and bring her into the barn.

At this point, intubation was needed, the process of inserting a tube from the mouth through the trachea, so that lung function could continue unobstructed. It required more courage than skill: Two men did the job, one to hold the mouth open, while the other crawled in with a head lamp and a very large endotracheal tube. Once in place, the end of the tube was attached to an equally impressive ventilator. Our patient was now ready for her operation.

The trunk was prepared and draped much like a human extremity, and we started the debridement process – the removal of damaged and useless material from the end of the trunk. Blood flowed so voluminously that we quickly, but belatedly, realized that a tourniquet was needed. The scrub clothes I was wearing were quickly saturated with elephant blood, and the macabre thought crossed my mind that if I were to be stopped in traffic on the way home I could well be accused of being an axe murderer.

Soon, though, everything was under control, and the simple reshaping of the trunk was fairly easily accomplished.

The lady recovered quickly, and we examined her carefully the next day during postoperative rounds. We immediately saw that we had greatly underestimated the elephant's adaptive capability. She was already eating hay without the use of a prehensile function, simply twirling her trunk around in the hay stack, just as a child gathers cotton candy on a stick.

A few days later, I returned to my oversized patient. She had already learned to eat chunks of elephant chow. This was another discovery for me; there really is such a thing as Purina Elephant Chow. It comes not in bags, but in dump trucks. The attendants had filled a large washtub with it, and our patient flexed her trunk into a hook shape to scoop food out of the tub.

One month later, I made my last follow-up visit. Cosmetically, the new tip was a great success. From the functional aspect, however, the reshaping had not been necessary, as the elephant had already learned how to manage food handling without the trunk's original grasping function. Nonetheless, we were able to persuade her to eat fresh grass, using the refashioned prehensile mechanism.

A happy outcome for our patient. I felt good that what had been entirely experimental and untried turned out so well.

As I drove away that last time from the zoo, my mind kept running through the old refrain:

Ellie the elephant's packed her trunk,
She's going to join the <u>cir</u>-cus...

COULDN'T BE DONE

ARIE FLEISCHER, M.D. BROOKLYN, NY

*"A man who has to be convinced to act before he acts
is not a man of action...you must act as you breathe."*
–Clemenceau

As a resident in plastic surgery, I had taken to heart the 'three A's, which were taught as being essential to successful practice – affability, availability, and ability. I recognized the wisdom of these axioms; one of them – availability – was to become crucial during my first few days in a major Brooklyn hospital.

One of the major attractions of that hospital was the small number of plastic surgeons on staff, implying plenty of opportunity to practice my chosen specialization. So when my name came over the loudspeakers requesting my presence in the operating room, I was happy, although not surprised. And of course I was available.

The surgeon who had initiated the call was the head of Oncology and the Head-and-Neck service. Once I was in the OR, he took a moment to explain the situation to me.

"This young woman," he said, indicating the prone figure on the operating table, "has developed a very advanced carcinoma of the thyroid gland – her previous treatment was probably inadequate – radiation therapy not aggressive enough."

He paused for a moment to have a few words with the anesthesiologist.

"We've had to do an emergency tracheostomy, as you can see," he continued. "This resectioning procedure will, of course, remove all the cancerous tissue. I've done a complete removal of the larynx, all the neck lymph glands, and left just one jugular vein. And I've taken out the windpipe to within about an inch of the lungs."

He put down the forceps he was holding. "She'll need to have the exposed neck vessels covered, and then we'll have to find a way to exteriorize that short tracheal stump. People need to breathe, you know. So, Arie – over to you."

With that, he turned and left the table.

Later, as I got to know him better, the surgeon and I became good friends. He was competent, he was aggressive; but, in this case, over-optimistic in evaluating the extent of the woman's malignancy. The amount of resectioning, of tissue removal, was very extensive, and I felt that he had not anticipated the challenge it presented to subsequent reconstructive surgery.

Over to me, indeed.

My background in the specialization was a solid one – a good residency training, with an aesthetic fellowship afterwards. However, one area in which my experience had been less focused was that of head-and-neck. The reason was that the usual practice at Presbyterian Hospital, where I trained, was for most of the head/neck malignancies and reconstructions after resection to be performed by the Ear, Nose, and Throat department. As a result, because I belonged to the Plastic Surgery department, my exposure to this type of procedure was adequate, but more limited.

I looked at the patient and felt overwhelmed by the challenges her case presented. There were more things missing from her than any other patient I had ever encountered. But there was no possibility of backing down. Reconstructive action was required immediately.

There came into my mind a saying from my native country, which is, "need is the best teacher." I decided to go ahead and do the best possible with the knowledge available to me.

First thing to be addressed was the trachea, the windpipe. It was far too short to be exteriorized in the orthodox way; I felt that an additional tube would be needed. It seemed logical to create a skin tube carried on a skin muscle flap of tissue with a blood supply at its base – in this case, using the pectoralis major muscle. I proceeded to raise this muscle flap and to have it carry a rectangle of skin formed into a tube. Then I transferred the flap into the mid-chest and neck, sutured the lower end of the tracheal stump, and brought the upper end to the skin at the front of the neck as a permanent tracheostomy.

I used the muscle to cover the exposed vessels, closed the donor site with a maneuver known as a Z-plasty, and neatly closed off all incisions in the best traditions of good plastic surgery to minimize noticeable scarring.

I was relieved and delighted when the patient made a good recovery and was eventually discharged from the hospital. But my more immediate reaction after the surgery was to make an intensive search of the available literature to find out how such a procedure was being carried out routinely – I hadn't had the opportunity to do this before being called into the OR.

What I learned was that the problem was rare, extremely difficult to handle, and the cumbersome procedures in general use were fraught with complications and inadequate results. A sudden revelation came to me: I had, in fact, invented a new operation. I submitted it as a case report, which was subsequently published.

Several years later, a patient with a similar problem came my way. I performed the same operation, with the same satisfactory results. I'm convinced that both patients were helped by this procedure, obviating the need for a mid-chest tracheostomy with its inherent risks and complications. It is a much better way of handling this rare set of circumstances.

The fact that I was successful in achieving a better outcome for these patients has more than a touch of irony. I was unprepared for the procedure I used. What I did was of course based on sound plastic surgery principles; but, because it had not been attempted before, there was no one to say that it couldn't or shouldn't be done. A strange way to learn, but it worked.

One of those rare occasions when ignorance is bliss.

PENILE PENALTIES

CHARLES E. HORTON, M.D.   NORFOLK, VA

*Care more for the individual patient than for
the special features of the disease.*
–Osler

In olden days, mostly in forgotten but warlike kingdoms, victorious generals would order their soldiers to cut off and collect the phalluses from vanquished (presumably dead!) foes, for presentation to their king or emperor. These baskets full of amputated penises would be dumped before the throne, and used to verify the count of the enemy dead.

This type of victory tally, the equivalent of today's only slightly less macabre "body count," has long been abandoned. However, surgery of the genital area has expanded: it is amazing to consider that circumcision has now become the most common surgery worldwide done for "cosmetic reasons. "

In my own forty-five year career as a genitourinary reconstructive surgeon, two cases with most unusual circumstances stand out in my mind. Let me recount them for you. Their extraordinary nature warrants the telling.

REDUCTION

A middle-aged physician came to me and asked that his penis be reduced in size. Before I examined him, he noted and commented on my skepticism. Unless he had penile lymphedema (and I had treated dozens of such cases) I had never heard of a patient <u>wanting</u> his penis to be smaller.

He assured me emphatically that he did not have lymphedema. The issue was simply that his penis was too large for him to have normal intercourse with his wife – lovemaking caused her pain, and their relationship was being destroyed. Even though he was a doctor, he had been unable to find anyone willing or able to reduce his swollen and distorted penis.

His medical history included an earlier episode of priapism, probably of sickle cell origin. His large penis had become enormously distended and swollen, and the internal blood channels were thrombosed and fibrous. The organ was now firm, more than fourteen inches long and as thick as a baseball.

After I had examined him, he said, "Now you can understand why intercourse would give my wife great pain." I nodded agreement.

The timing of his complaint was fortunate; we had been working on techniques for reconstruction of the tunica albuginea, the lining of the normal blood spaces of the penis. I explained this to him, and outlined the procedure that I would recommend.

He agreed, and we went ahead with the operation. His penis was shortened by excisional surgery, preserving the nerve supply and sensation. The circumference of the organ was reduced to less than that of a billiard ball.

My patient/physician healed well, and was overjoyed at the result. Subsequently he reported that his wife was much more relieved, and very happy, and I assumed that their marital relationship was back on an even keel.

There was no description in the literature about penile reduction operations, but we were able to apply the well-established principles of plastic surgery to the problem and achieve a successful result. The specialty of plastic surgery is noted for its innovative and creative approaches to unusual and perplexing circumstances, and for achieving by these methods surprisingly good outcomes.

REMOVAL

A husband and wife came together to see me with a most unusual request to cut off his penis.

Obviously, I needed to dig deeply into the background of this question before coming to any conclusions. I had a long discussion with both of them, during which it transpired that three years earlier he had been hunting. His shotgun had accidentally fired, peppering his groin and penile area with multiple pellets. After that incident, he had continuous severe pain in his penis, and had undergone five operations to cut nerves, and to remove pellets and scars. In spite of all this surgery, however, the pain remained constant and close to unbearable.

He and his wife ran a small business. The pain he suffered was interfering badly with his management skills, to the extent that the enterprise was going downhill so fast that they were on the verge of declaring bankruptcy. In front of me, they frankly acknowledged their love for each other. Then the wife told me that she would be prepared to forego all sexual activities if only he could be relieved of the constant pain.

It was evident that more depended on the help that might be available for this man than simply the relief of his pain. Without such relief, their business would fail, their finances would be in ruins, and the education of their children would be in jeopardy.

To complete the diagnostic picture, I sent my patient to a psychiatrist, a neurologist, and a pain center. All three verified the reality of the perceived pain. They agreed that it had been properly addressed at university clinics, and that all treatments had failed.

I considered all this information with great care. When the patient came into my office again, I instructed him to contine to take the prescribed medications. I told him of the possibility of "phantom pain," that strange phenomenon by which pain can be felt even after its source has been amputated, and recommended that he return to his psychiatrist to assess that possibility in his case.

Three months went by. The couple reappeared in my office, again begging for surgery. Again, I advised delay before making a final, irrevocable decision, and sent them back to the neurologist and the pain clinic.

Another three months. They called for an emergency meeting with me. His words were chilling. "I've lost my business, I cannot work, and no one will help. Why won't you operate?

"My wife completely agrees and supports me in this decision. If nothing is done, I'm going to kill myself."

So after final heart-searching, and with all consultants in agreement, we removed as much of the scarring in both groins as possible. We released some, but not all, of the scars surrounding the many delicate nerves of the area, and finally amputated his penis. The procedure was successfully completed. The patient healed uneventfully, and on discharge from the hospital, he told us that the constant severe pain was gone. He returned home to be cared for by his local physician and to have psychiatric support, while we anxiously waited to hear the long-term benefits of his surgery.

Several months later, his wife called to report that her husband was still pain-free, and that they were reviving the business. Three months on, she telephoned again, this time to say, "Thank you for giving me back my husband! "

Obviously things were working out as they had hoped. Another three years went by, and then I received a call from husband and wife together.

"Dr. Horton, our business is progressing well, and we are very happy. What you did was the only thing in the world to help us. A simple "thank you" is too little to say – but we mean it most sincerely."

In a different case such as this – more difficult perhaps in its ethical dimension even than in the surgery involved – a doctor goes through mental anguish in trying to make the right decision, an anguish the nonmedical public can never appreciate. Fortunately, in this case the decision was the right one, and the results clearly affirm that.

But in dealing with the complexities of the human body, we simple physicians cannot always predict the outcomes. If this surgery had not been as successful as it turned out to be, this story might have been stained with tears of sorrow.

EXCELLENCE IS WHERE YOU FIND IT

DAVID W. FUNAS, M.D. ORANGE, CA

"A problem is a chance for you to do your best."

–Duke Ellington

He was a perfect poster boy for a fund-raising brochure. Just three months old, the child exhibited a wide, complete, unilateral cleft lip. I had come to the end of my Tuesday session at Leon's University Hospital, Nicaragua, a single-story building with a rusty corrugated iron roof. I wrote the baby boy's name on my calendar as the first case for my schedule in the Leon operating room, and asked the staff to make sure that time was held.

The year was 1966, and I was serving as a doctor on the *SS Hope*, the ex-World War II hospital ship which had been converted into a center for medical treatment and training to benefit third world countries. The vessel was anchored off Corinto, Nicaragua's main port. After I had left the Leon hospital, I went onboard and operated on the ship for two days. Then off again, this time to Hospital Adventista in the mountains of Chinandega.

A few days later, a VW bus took our team back to Leon. I was anticipating the challenge and the gratification of correcting a wide cleft lip with a Millard rotation-advancement closure. But, when we arrived, I was surprised to be told by the chief surgical resident that my operating schedule had been rearranged. We would start with what had been previously scheduled as the second case. The parents of my patient had decided not to wait, and a Nicaraguan surgeon had performed the closure instead. The baby was ready for suture removal and discharge the next day.

166

Nicaragua is a country where something amazing happens every day. Today's feature was the lack of sophistication of a family who would not wait a week for a Board Certified Associate Professor of Surgery (Plastic) from the United States of America to perform his artistry on their baby, and to demonstrate the artistry to the Nicaraguan doctors.

Still, I felt I had not lost the opportunity to further educate these doctors in their medical and surgical skills by critiquing the operation which had been carried out.

I took my retinue of staff, residents, and students to the child in his crib. I scanned the lip to determine what point was the most important error with which to open my critique.

Cupid's bow? . . . no, it was horizontal, precisely positioned.

Columellar asymmetry, of course . . . no, it was almost perfectly symmetrical.

I knew that the nostril floor would be wide, because it was a Tennison repair . . . nonetheless, the nostrils were as symmetrical as my "Millard" nostrils.

The sutures were black silk, a material I have always considered to be crude – I use synthetic monofilament materials. I would cover important points in suturcraft. But wait a minute. I inspected the fine 6-0 silk sutures more closely. The tension was just right. The closure was beautiful.

I stood silent. The group around me was listening expectantly for my words of surgical wisdom. Finally, I spoke.

"I thought that there were no plastic surgeons in Nicaragua."

"No hay."
"Who closed this baby's cleft?"
"Dr. Melendez, el cirugano pediatrico."

I couldn't find out anything more about Dr. Melendez, except that he was a very busy, young pediatric surgeon who worked in many places on many children.

The only way I could think of to end the "teaching" session was to congratulate the parents on their handsome boy.

CREDIT WHERE CREDIT IS DUE?

ENRIQUE A. PASARELL, M.D.
SAN JUAN, PUERTO RICO

Experience is not what happens to a man,
it is what a man does with what happens to him.
–Aldous Huxley

I was training in Indianapolis under my professor, Jim Bennet, M.D., when I encountered a situation from which I learned an important lesson: human perception, human trust, and human prejudice are interlinked phenomena.

An English teenage girl was admitted to our children's hospital for burn scar revision of her face. I was the intern, so the admission history and physical examination were my responsibilities. The young lady's mother was with her, and during the interview she asked me quite pointedly who would be performing the operation.

I was not sure why she had asked the question, although obviously it had been triggered by either my inexperience or my strong Hispanic accent. But as the girl was one of Dr. Bennet's private patients, I had no hesitation in responding "Dr. Bennet, of course."

On the day of the surgery, Dr. Bennett handed me the scalpel. During the entire operation, he took on the roles of professor and assistant, while I carried out the procedure. I did a complete resurfacing of the forehead with a split thickness skin graft, a hair-bearing free scalp graft to one of the eyebrows, and scar revision of the eyelids.

Later, when the dressings came off, the mother was surprised and really excited to see the immediate improvement.

Suddenly more aware than I had previously been of the link-age – perception/prejudice/trust – I made just one remark.

"Yes, ma'am, the man is a genius!"

ENOUGH IS ENOUGH

ENRIQUE A. PASARELL, M.D.
SAN JUAN, PUERTO RICO

The difficulty in life is the choice.
–George Moore

The young lady who came into my private practice some time back was petite, attractive, and intelligent. When I say "petite" I really mean quite tiny – she was less than five feet tall, and weighed only a hundred pounds.

She wanted evaluation and advice on the damage which two pregnancies and lactation had inflicted on her body. I examined her, and then reviewed for her the possibilities of mastopexy and abdominoplasty. She listened carefully, never interrupting. It was clear that she understood my explanations, so I was surprised by the question she asked when I'd finished.

"Doctor," she asked, "do you perform penile enlargement?"

Swiftly following the new direction she had taken, I pointed out to her that this type of surgery is very controversial, and that it does not add any length to the penis.

Her comment was quick and clear. "Oh, length is no problem. We have measured it, and his is nine inches long."

She stood up, expressed her appreciation for my explanations and my sincere approach to her problems, and left my office. From that day to this, we have never again met.

Some people are never satisfied!

STREAMLINED FOR SUCCESS

FREDRICK LUKASH, M.D.   MANHASSET, NY

Genuine responsibility exists only where there is real responding.
—Buber

I do a lot of pediatric and adolescent plastic surgery. One of the unique things that I do is have all the children I operate on draw me pictures of their before and after experiences. I was written up in the *New York Times* regarding an art exhibit of these works.

I received a phone call from a distraught woman whose grandson lived in Florida and was suffering from a bilateral prominent ear deformity. The ears were huge, and the child was psychologically stigmatized. He was on anti-psychotic medications and was retreating into himself to the point of almost being considered autistic. The psychological profile of this child was presented to the Florida Medical Board, who agreed that bilateral otoplasty (pinning back the ears) would be of benefit. However, this child belonged to an HMO, which refused to pay for this surgery in spite of the medical board's recommendation. The grandmother contacted me and asked if I would be of service. I volunteered to do the surgery at no compensation if they could bring the child to New York.

The child underwent a successful otoplasty as an outpatient, spent the week in New York with his grandmother, and then returned to Florida. Follow-up letters and photographs from the family revealed that this child was out of his shell, off all medications, and acting like a normal teenager.

172

THE ENGLISH PATIENT

JACOB GOLAN, M.D. JERUSALEM, ISRAEL

I promise to be sincere, but not to be impartial.
–Goethe

When I was a young surgeon, I decided to travel internationally to learn new and improved techniques, a common practice among surgeons everywhere. So I went to England, where I spent most of my time in a big university center in London. Every Monday, however, I took advantage of an opportunity to observe a famous British plastic surgeon who had a private practice in the capital. After a while, we became good friends. I look back on those Mondays with appreciation, and with the memory of how much I enjoyed my time with him.

One week, however, things were not the same. He was nervous and irritable, but I had no idea why. Finally, he put this edginess into words.

"Jacob, you'll have to excuse me, but I just can't have you here next Monday. Go and find something to do. Go shopping, do anything you wish . . . just don't come on Monday."

Of course I stayed away that Monday, but I was still totally unaware of what lay behind this embargo. I felt that it must have been something of great importance to him; he was usually a model of quiet British reserve, and this display of worried nervousness was quite out of character for him.

The following Monday, we were back together again. He seemed completely relieved of whatever burden had been troubling him, and he resumed his usual unflustered personality. He didn't mention his prohibition on my being there the previous week, and I didn't bring the subject up.

Months later, it was time for me to return home. I went to his office to thank him and say my farewells. He said, "Sit down a minute, I want to tell you what was really happening on the Monday when I didn't want you here." I waited, my curiosity aroused.

He went on, "My daughter needed breast reduction surgery. Common practice, as you well know, is to let one's colleagues perform an operation on a relative. But I thought it over, kept running it through my mind, and I couldn't help remembering the scars that some of them had left on their patients. So I decided to shun tradition, and to do the operation myself."

So now I knew. He had made an unusual decision, but having carried it through on that memorable Monday, all the anxiety that had been making him a nervous wreck disappeared. Whether the operation was a good one, or if his daughter ended up with less visible scarring than his colleagues used to leave at that stage of plastic surgery development, I don't know.

I shall never know . . . .

THE SICK MAN

JACOB GOLAN, M.D. JERUSALEM, ISRAEL

*There is but an inch of difference between the
cushioned chambers and the padded cell.*
–Chesterton

She was a relatively young woman who sat before me, and her voice was charged with anxiety. Easily understandable; her beloved but much older husband had undergone coronary bypass surgery just a few days before. He had come through the operation successfully, although he'd been very sick beforehand.

Now he had a new problem, myelitis of the sternum - inflammation of the marrow of the breastbone – a condition which flashed red danger lights. His cardiac surgeons believed they should delay the procedure to clean and repair the infected sternum for a day or two, to give time for his situation to stabilize. My own staff agreed with the heart specialists.

"Doctor," said the wife, obviously extremely worried, "I must beg you to help me by making sure that this second operation is done just as soon as possible." She stopped speaking, dabbed her eyes with a handkerchief, and took a deep breath before going on. "I love him so much, and I couldn't bear the thought of losing him. I'd never forgive myself if I hadn't done everything I could for him to have this life-saving operation."

I was touched by her intense concern for the well-being of

her husband, and, in spite of its being a weekend, we decided to operate on the old man right away. The surgical team was assembled, the procedure was performed by one of my staff members, and everything went very well.

I put the whole episode out of my mind until a week or so later, when I asked the surgeons and my own staff people what had happened to the patient and his worried young wife after the successful outcome of his serious condition.

The man, I was told, was doing extremely well. The young woman, on the other hand, was a different story. When she found that her cherished husband did not die, she disappeared. That's it. Gone. Nowhere to be found.

It took some time before it came to light that she had a young lover, and that she had hoped that the much older man would not survive the second operation.

None of us were sorry that we had disappointed her. On the contrary, we were only too glad that our surgical skills had been able to pull our patient through a dangerous set of circumstances.

UNSPEAKABLE GRATITUDE

JAMES E. VOGEL, M.D.   BALTIMORE, MD

Most men cry better than they speak.
–Thoreau

This has to do with a 25-year-old woman, who had a very significant bump on the nose. In addition, the nasal tip was drooping, plunging inferiorly, and she had a very small chin. She had always been teased about her witch-like appearance and it bothered her considerably. We had a consultation to discuss the surgery that would improve her appearance. She then went on to have a rhinoplasty and chin augmentation.

After seven days, she returned to the office and we took the splint off her nose and removed the tapes from her chin. She had a marvelous result. When she saw herself in the mirror and assessed her profile, she was so incredibly happy that she broke down in tears. She was so emotional, she couldn't talk and she had to reschedule her follow-up appointment for the next day.

The improvement in this woman's self-esteem and her new level of confidence were extremely gratifying to see. The experience stands out in my mind as one of the most rewarding cosmetic surgery procedures I have performed.

REVERSED ROLES

ROGER SALISBURY, M.D.   VALHALLA, NY

A man never reveals his character more vividly
than when portraying the character of another.
                    –Richter

The Army Burn Center was one of a very small number of such specialized units in the United States in the early 1970s. Many areas of the country were underserved in terms of rapid responses to severe burn injuries; so as a result, we often flew civilian emergency missions as well as carrying out the military evacuation function.

If we were summoned by a call within a two-hundred mile radius, one of our own rescue helicopters would pick us up at the hospital's helipad, fly us to the site, and bring us back with the injured person. Calls farther away would be handled by means of an Air Force jet which would take a burn surgeon and a Corpsman, together with their "burn chest," to the emergency.

One eventful day, a call came from south Texas. We jumped aboard the helicopter and took off to collect the burned patient. When we arrived, I found the woman to be in respiratory distress, and I had to do an emergency tracheotomy.

That procedure completed, we gently got her into the aircraft and quickly became airborne. So far, so good. But, within a few minutes, the next emergency developed. Our rotor malfunctioned, and down we went, like a stone. Our pilot switched to auto-rotation, which slowed our scary descent

178

somewhat, and then had time to get off a quick mayday with our position.

Only one thought went through my mind as we headed earthward, still at breakneck speed: I was destined to be burned and admitted to my own unit. That prospect held little charm for me.

In any event, we did not explode when we hit the ground. Still, we were all badly shaken and could do little except sit on the grass and wait for help.

After twenty minutes, we saw two helicopters approaching from the direction of San Antonio. They landed in close formation in the field next to where our damaged aircraft lay, tilted to one side. I jumped up and ran toward the lead chopper. I could see that the pilot was waving frantically at me, but because his smoke visor was still down I could not identify a face.

As his rotor stopped, I moved in closer. The door opened, the pilot leaned out and pushed up his visor.

"Hey, Doc! How ya doin'?"

I was stunned beyond speech. I was looking into the face of an ex-patient of the Burn Center, a pilot who, in trying to evade hostile gunfire, had crashed into a mountainside in Vietnam. He had been terribly burned, but after many months of care in the Center and subsequent rehabilitation, he made a full recovery.

Mike Petersen had been one of our favorite patients. A wonderful, clever man, a college graduate, married to a school teacher, he was an outstanding pilot in Vietnam. Clearly, he had been destined to continue his aviation career, but he represented a problem to the military – to them, it appeared unlikely that after such devastating injuries he could resume active duty.

We in the Center viewed it differently. We felt that the whole process of rehabilitation was to restore him to his pre-injury status, and we pushed this concept through the command channels, using him as a test case. We prevailed. And now here he was, rescuing us.

As our lady patient was being transferred into the other helicopter, Mike called out again. "Great to see ya, Doc! Climb on board!"

My reply was instinctive.

"Climb aboard, my ass! I know how bad a pilot you are! You <u>flew</u> into the side of a mountain in Vietnam – we only <u>crashed</u> here in Texas! No, thanks, I'll take a cab back to the hospital."

He loved it. Our flight back to San Antonio was uneventful.

We've had many laughs about this incident when we have met up over the years. But beyond the funny side of this apparent coincidence, it seems to me that life does have a certain symmetry. It was, I believe, entirely appropriate that Mike Petersen, having once been so close to death, was granted the opportunity not only to fly again, but to help those who had once helped him.

ONLY MY JOB

SAMEER I. SHEHADI, M.D.
BEIRUT, LEBANON

We can do noble acts without ruling earth and sea.
–Aristotle

West Beirut, 1977. The Lebanese civil war had been raging for more than a year. The surgical facilities of the American University Hospital were in danger of being overwhelmed by the never-ending flow of casualties.

I was chairman of the Department of Surgery, as well as being the only plastic surgeon in the city, and it fell to me to make the difficult decision to suspend all elective admissions and to handle only nontransferable emergencies. To ensure strict adherence to this war-caused policy, I checked every casualty that came to the emergency department and made a personal decision on who was to be admitted.

Early one morning, I was called to make decisions about a batch of wounded people who had just arrived. I had three options: The most severe cases would go directly to the operating room; the next group would go to a holding area to await surgery; and the least serious would be treated and discharged.

I had completed the triage process for all but one, a young man perhaps twenty years of age, who had a minor soft tissue injury to his leg. I directed the resident to clean up the wound and then to discharge him.

Hearing these instructions, the patient suddenly sat up on his stretcher, pulled out a pistol from his clothes, and pointed it a few inches from my head. "You have to admit me."

To this day, I can recall vividly that gun as I saw it from the corner of my eye. I froze, and broke into a cold sweat. To run and take cover was not an option, as I calculated that any sudden move might cause him to panic and pull the trigger.

It was like a still from a movie and lasted for perhaps a minute, although to me it was eternity. Totally unexpectedly, rescue came in the form of the nursing supervisor. She swooped from behind me, put her arm over my shoulders, and in a flash of violent movement shoved my resident and me into the radiology dark room, the nearest doorway in the OR.

She slammed the door shut, yelling, "Stay until I come back." We were left in complete darkness. We could hear screaming and shouting, and then an eerie silence. We were safe.

Several months passed, but the fighting continued. Triage had become a familiar routine.

I was called upon once more to make decisions about a new group of casualties. With a shock of recognition, I saw that one of them was the same young man who had threatened my life earlier. He was in no shape to see who I was, as he had a serious abdominal injury.

I operated on him to close the wound. He made good progress; there was no postoperative infection, and the damage repaired itself well. As healing went on, I saw him several times when I made my daily rounds or monitored his recovery. On these occasions, he was always subdued and distant, and rarely looked me in the face.

Eventually, it was time for him to leave the hospital. I went to check him and to give him his discharge instructions. As I was leaving, he looked up."You did not recognize me."

I stopped, and turned to face him. "Of course I did. You are the guy who pointed a gun to my head not long ago."

His face turned red. He tried to grab my hand and kiss it. "I am not fit to kiss your feet, and yet you operated on me and saved my life!"

I pulled my hand away from him and patted him on the back. "I was only doing my job."

THE GREAT CIRCLE

SAMEER I. SHEHADI, M.D.
BEIRUT, LEBANON

The luck of having talent is not enough;
one must also have a talent for luck.
            –Berlioz

I had just started my second year of residency in plastic surgery at St. Louis University, when I admitted Casey, a 65-year-old man suffering from skin cancer which had invaded all of his lower lip. Using orthodox procedures, the cancerous tissue was excised, and the lip reconstructed with flaps of skin.

That was only the beginning. Six months later, Casey was readmitted, this time with a large tumor fixed to the under-surface of his jaw and to the overlying skin.

Again I prepared him for an operation, which would consist of a radical dissection of the left side of his neck, and excision of the tumor with its involved skin.

I was scrubbing before the surgery when the attending surgeon turned to me.

"Sameer, I'd like to do this procedure – it could take a long time, and I want to be sure and finish in time for a television interview I've been asked to do at three this afternoon. Can't risk being late."

Then to work. The surgery went well, but it took longer than

184

we had expected to work our way around the tumor and separate it from the jaw we included the layer covering the bone with the specimen. We continued with the rest of the neck dissection, and I got the sense that the procedure was being hurried. The surgeon kept glancing at the clock. Obviously, the TV interview was on his mind.

As first assistant, it was my responsibility to keep pace with the surgeon, to anticipate his every next move, and – most important – to keep out of trouble. The operating room became quiet, and I could sense the tension in the air. Like the rest of the OR team, I remained silent and calculated the odds on finishing the surgery in time.

2:30 PM: The specimen came out, and the feeling of relief was palpable. The attending surgeon pulled the neck flaps together.

"Sameer, you can close this!"

And he was gone.

I was aware that the situation was a difficult and demanding one, but it wasn't until I completed suturing the neck flaps of skin that I appreciated its full complexity. There was a two-inch segment of bare jaw exposed in the upper neck. Pulling the flaps upward would cover the jaw, but also expose the carotid artery in the lower neck.

I hadn't heard the phrase "between a rock and hard place," but that is certainly where I now found myself. I decided that priority should be given to protecting the carotid artery.

I stopped to think what should be done next. I had no fallback adviser: He was already on television, and incommunicado.

Instinct made me reach for the knife (cautery in my resident days was taboo). I detached the origin of a neck muscle, tucked it under the cheek flap. Then I applied a split thickness skin graft over the muscle to complete the closure.

The source of blood supply to the muscle was the last thing on my mind; worse, I didn't bother to check it out later. This was 1962, at least ten years before muscle flaps were described.

Two days went by. The attending surgeon came by for his rounds, and casually asked to see our patient and to change his dressing. I felt more than a little anxious, and my hands were shaking as I exposed the dressing.

To my surprise and delight, the graft was fine, blood circulation was good, and it had "taken" completely.

"How did you cover the mandible?" I had expected this question from my boss.

I explained what I had done and why I had done it. He checked the patient's neck once more, nodded his approval.

"Good job, Shehadi!"

I was relieved, triumphant, proud. Even as the pent-up emotion swept over me, I was aware that my success did not escape Casey, who was watching the whole scene.

That's not the end of the story.

Twenty-two years went by. I returned to St. Louis University as Professor and Director of the Division of Plastic Surgery. Before I had even settled into my new office,

I got a call from Oncology, asking if I could come to see an old patient of mine.

I was surprised. I asked if this were a consultation, as I had not yet been granted my privileges.

"No. You operated on this patient's lip some time ago, and we are treating him for a second tumor. He asked to see you."

Instant flashback, "Is that Casey?" I asked – but I knew it was.

I went straight to the Oncology office, where Casey was expecting me, with a great beaming smile on his elderly and beautiful face. He gave me a big hug, and explained that he had read in the newspaper that I had returned to St. Louis, and that he wanted to say hi.

He winked, and added, "I knew you would be a big shot one day!"

I walked back to my office. My eyes were damp, but I had a wonderful feeling in my heart.

Chapter VI
Empowerment

A FAREWELL TO CRIME

BRUNNO RISTOW, M.D.
SAN FRANCISCO, CA

*The universe is transformation; our life is what
our thoughts make it.*
–Marcus Aurelius Antoninus

It was a rainy day in San Francisco not long ago when I first met Mrs. Winter (not her real name, of course). She was accompanied by her husband, and she had come for a consultation about the possibilities for facial rejuvenation.

Mrs. Winter was a woman of remarkably serious appearance. Her skin was "indoor pale," she had blue eyes and chestnut hair, and wore a gray suit of formal cut. Her brow was permanently frown-furrowed; her lips were thin and tight, slightly turned down at the corners. She was clearly a no-nonsense type of personality.

I had read her chart before the couple came into the office, and her career background matched the impression she made. She was a field agent involved in major investigations into financial crime in international markets, working for the U.S. government's main criminal division in Washington, D.C. When we got into general discussion, she revealed that she carried a 9mm pistol at all times and was extremely proficient at its use.

Her husband was well-educated, well-dressed, and active in West Coast financial markets. We talked about the projected rejuvenation procedure, and he was quite open in saying that he supported, but did not encourage, her desires in this area. The rest of the consultation was unexciting. It consisted of my explanation of the course of action I proposed and her agreement with that.

Some time later, I carried out a facelift, to include work on the much-lined forehead, the neck, and around the eyes. Dermabrasion improved her skin texture, and volume restoration of upper and lower lips was designed to lessen her appearance of such grim seriousness.

A month later, Mrs. Winter came back alone for a follow-up visit. It was a transformation scene. Her make-up was perfectly applied; her suit was a knit celadon green wool with gold braid accents, very much like one of the more discrete Chanel designs; her shoes perfectly complemented the ensemble.

She met me with an engaging smile, and her whole face lit up to radiate a completely different personalty – warm, friendly, happy.

"And how," I could not refrain from asking, "is the business of criminal investigation in the United States government?"

"Oh, tomorrow is my last day. I quit, Dr. Ristow! It's a new beginning for me. I'm going to decorating school."

I suppose I should have been more surprised than I was, but I had experienced this sort of life-change many times before. Aesthetic surgery can be a powerful catalyst.

CHANGE OF DIET

MIRIAM HAREL, M.D.
FRAMINGHAM, MA

The bosom-weight, your stubborn gift,
that no philosophy can lift.
—William Wadsworth

Plastic surgeons know that reduction/mammoplasty patients – women who elect to have this procedure for smaller breasts – are the most grateful patients they have. For this reason, I like to do this operation more than any other.

One of my patients was a lady in her sixties. She came to me for the procedure to be performed because the size of her bosom was a continuing embarrassment to her. We agreed on a date to go ahead, and her attitude can only be described as enthusiastic.

The operation went through with no complications. She handled the postoperative phase comfortably and then visited me again in my office.

"How are you feeling?" I asked her, although I could see from her smiling face that she was happy – ecstatic, even – with the result. Her reply was a picturesque comment that has stuck in my mind ever since.

"Oh, I feel wonderful. It's the first time in my life that I didn't have boobs for lunch!"

A memorable and amusing summing-up of her new take on life.

NOSE JOB

PETER R. NEUMANN, M.D.
GREAT NECK, NY

Virtue is bold, and goodness never fearful.
—William Shakespeare
"Measure for Measure," Act III

One cold and blustery night, back in the early '70s, I had my dramatic introduction to plastic surgery. I was an intern, a first-year general surgery resident, and I found myself in charge of the emergency room in Buffalo General Hospital.

The inner-city area of Buffalo tended to display a great deal of violent behavior, but as the evening wore on, things were relatively quiet. The ER was an oasis of calm, and we sat around munching on chicken wings and talking about future parties that we had planned.

The peacefulness was shattered by the shrill ringing of the red telephone. The call was to let us know that there had been a fight between two rival gangs in town, resulting in many injury cases of varying degrees of severity.

We began to mobilize. The wintry conditions outside had left four feet of snow on the ground, so we knew we had to give staff outside the hospital, as well as those in the buildings, as much advance information as we could concerning the developing situation in the ER. We called attending surgeons, interns, and residents in several specialties, and put them on notice, telling them that we would call for them when patients started arriving.

Twelve minutes after the red telephone had sounded the alarm, the first ambulance pulled up – there would be fourteen by the time they had all reached us. Many of them had more than one injury case. As well as the fleet of ambulances, sixteen police cars – lights flashing, sirens wailing – arrived on the scene. It turned out that nearly all of these wounded "warriors" were under arrest. The first casualties to stumble in were on foot, exhibiting a variety of lacerations, contusions, and abrasions. One had been stabbed in the back with a short knife; he went into a major trauma room. Several had broken arms and legs, and they were put into the holding areas to wait for the orthopedists.

I was especially impressed with the sheer size and appearance of one of the casualties. Standing six feet four inches, weighing some 285 pounds, and sporting an enormous beard, he had one hand handcuffed to his belt while the other held a towel to his face. He was accompanied by two policemen, one on each side.

He came up to me, as I was acting as triage doctor, and spoke in a voice muffled by the towel.

"Doc, they bit it off."

I wasn't too sure of what he had said, as the voice from behind the towel was difficult to make out against the general clamor. He lowered the towel from his face, draped it over his shoulder, and clumsily groped in his pocket. He pulled out a crumpled handkerchief and spoke again.

"Here, Doc, this is for you." He handed me the soiled and bloody rag. In it was his nose.

He had been in a fight in which his opponent had bitten it

off, including all the cartilaginous portion. When I looked up at this face, I saw that the only parts remaining were the two nasal bones and the nasal spine.

I turned at once to the young student nurse standing next to me, handed her the nose, and made the mistake of being light-hearted about the wound.

"Nurse, go get this cloned" I said, referring to a Woody Allen movie current at the time. She immediately became almost hysterical, and dropped the nose on the floor. The head nurse saw what had happened, picked up the nose, and took both it and the patient – and the two policemen – into a back room.

When all the other patients had been triaged and taken care of, I went to the room to see the patient. He was lying there, peaceful and relaxed – unusually so, considering the circumstances.

"Doc," he said, "I know that this nose is going to work out."

"I'm going to call the plastic surgeon for you," I replied, "and have him reattach your nose."

He looked hard at me. "You're my doctor – you're reattaching my nose."

By now the time was 2:30 a.m. I called the plastic surgery resident and explained the situation to him. He was less than cooperative.

"The snow's piled up outside, my baby has the flu, my wife has been crabby . . . if this character wants you as his doctor, you ARE his doctor. Sew it back on." Click. He hung up on me.

So – back to the patient. I spent the rest of the night re-attaching the nose in multiple layers, using whatever knowledge I had – at that stage, not much. We first washed it in pHisoHex, cleaned up the nonviable edges, then sewed back the tissue using chromic and nylons, the materials of that time. It was seven in the morning by the time we finished and, although I was bone-tired, I felt that I'd done a wonderful job.

Later that day, the plastic surgery chief resident came in on rounds. He pointed to my friend with the reattached nose.

"Look what our newest plastic surgery fellow has just done!"

When the chief attending surgeon found out that the operation had been performed by a mere first-year resident, he hit the roof. But despite that, I will always remember that the episode was my introduction to my specialization of plastic surgery.

As a footnote, the nose survived almost completely, the only exception being a small distal portion which the plastic surgery resident eventually debrided and put on a pinch graft. I never saw the patient again.

BELOW THE SURFACE

ROGER SIMPSON, M.D. GARDEN CITY, NY

There are more things in heaven and earth . . .
Than are dreamt of in your philosophy.
—William Shakespeare

As director of a plastic surgery residency program, it is my annual responsibility to interview candidates. Those interviews invariably reveal that the candidates take deeply to heart one opportunity above all others: the potential ability to use their skills to change people's lives.

I well remember that emotion when I started in the specialization. And today, despite the pressures of a busy practice, I still encounter patients and situations who startlingly reaffirm its reality. That reality may at times be hidden, but occasionally it bursts out like the sun from behind a storm cloud. Such a case was that of a woman I'll call Mary.

Before the nurse brought Mary into my office for consultation, I read through her chart. The laconically expressed complaint was "desires breast surgery." Her occupation was that of nurse with responsibility for the care of patients on a medical/surgical floor. She was forty-three years old.

She was shown in. After the introductions, I formed a first impression from the way she sat with her head downcast and her long, stringy hair unkempt, of a mild-mannered, almost meek person who cared little for her appearance. When she spoke, this impression was confirmed; her voice was so soft that I found it difficult to hear what she was saying.

With reluctant timidity, she told me that she was in my office to discuss the possibility of breast augmentation, but quickly apologized for even being interested in such a procedure.

She went on to say that while sitting in my waiting room, she had believed that she was among people who needed my attention more. She added that she felt extremely awkward talking about the possibility of such surgery.

Mary seemed to be a shy, almost shrinking personality type, who must have summoned all her courage just to talk with me.

I gently prompted her to tell me what she would like to have done.

"I've always wanted to have more . . . more form to my breasts." Her voice was even quieter now. "When I was an adolescent, my bosom just didn't seem to grow like other girls'. I've always been embarrassed whatever clothes I wear, and often I put on more layers of clothing just to hide my childish figure."

"Well," I said, "there are a lot of young ladies who face the same situation. I want to assure you that surgery can help you make the best of yourself. Let me examine you." I called in my nurse.

My examination confirmed that for a woman of her height – five feet seven inches – her breast development was indeed minimal. She put her clothes on again and sat down – still with the same dejected attitude.

"Doctor, I want you to understand that I only want the smallest augmentation – nothing with any fullness, and certainly nothing that my friends could connect to this procedure. I'm still embarrassed merely discussing it, and the most I want is to fill an A-cup bra." She swallowed, then went on. "You do understand, don't you, doctor?"

One of the most fascinating aspects of plastic surgery is that it gives the practitioner an insight, a sort of psychological window, into peoples' lives and their inner thoughts. Intuitively, I suspected that this woman's desire was far greater than anything she'd expressed.

With my nurse still in the room, we talked for several minutes about the technicalities of such a procedure, about scheduling, about recovery times. Being a nurse herself, my prospective patient had a good understanding of these issues and was able progressively to relate to me more, if only on a professional level.

I assessed that this conversation had given her increased confidence in my judgement – enough confidence for me to suggest that she might want to consider a larger augmentation than she was presently thinking of.

Mary moved uneasily in her chair. "I don't really know what that would do for me, doctor. Perhaps it wouldn't be in my own best interests."

"Let me try something." I turned to my nurse and asked her to bring in a larger-cup bra and fill it with 350cc gel implants. "Now hold the bra in place, and look at yourself in the mirror."

It was a transformation scene. This unimpressive woman

suddenly stood upright, squared her shoulders, and threw her hair back. She looked at herself from all angles, eyes aglow. Unable to tear away from her own reflection, she said:

"Can you really do this for me?"

"Yes."

She spun away from the mirror, swept off her wire-rimmed glasses in a dramatic gesture, and in a loud and clear voice exclaimed "Doctor, forget what I told you before. THIS is what I really want."

It took little time to make all the arrangements for the procedure to be carried out. It was fully successful and made reality of that transforming reflection in the mirror.

I saw Mary several times over a number of years. She had changed virtually overnight into a self-confident and attractive woman, outgoing and popular. Gone was the rather sad and sorry person who had come into my office with such low expectations. She had found herself, her real self.

I recognize my good fortune in being the agent of that revelation. Now, when I talk with our annual group of candidates and sense their desire to change lives, I recall Mary and smile.

SWEET REVENGE

S. ANTHONY WOLFE, M.D.
MIAMI, FL

*Logic and consistency are luxuries for the gods
and the lower animals.*
– Samuel Butler II

A number of years ago, a lady came in for a consultation about having a facelift. She was not beautiful to begin with; she had a very high forehead, low brows, a beak of a nose, and a bird face without much of a chin. On top of that, the aging process had not been kind to her. She said she had gotten divorced recently and that her ex-husband had repeatedly told her she was so ugly she should wear a bag over her head. She looked at me and said, "and you know, he was right . . . ."

We worked out a fairly ambitious operative plan which included a forehead lift, a rhinoplasty, a facelift and submental lipectomy, and a genioplasty. Everything went well, and all these procedures dramatically changed the overall shape, form, and appearance of her face. The brows were up, the nose was straight, the chin was proud, and the neck and all the slack in the face had been tightened up.

She came by several months later and told me that she had gone into the liquor store that her ex-husband owned. He didn't recognize her and, in fact, had tried to pick her up!

I think at least from her point of view, the outcome of this operation had been successful.

200

FAIRY TALES CAN COME TRUE

WILLIAM H. FRAZIER, M.D.
VERO BEACH, FL

Love slays what we have been that we may be what we were not.
–Saint Augustine

This is a story about a woman, divorced, in her mid-40s. She was a librarian in a small town in Connecticut. I had seen her teenaged daughter for evaluation and treatment of a prominent nose. She underwent nasoplasty and chin implant, had a great result, and went off to college, where she was both socially and academically successful. The mother, perhaps seeing herself in the daughter, thought that she, too, would benefit trom a similar procedure.

When I talked with her about her expectations, she said quite frankly that she was in a dead-end position in a small town. What she wanted was to get out of the environment, develop a more exciting life, and "marry a millionaire." I explained that cosmetic surgery would not ensure social success and definitely would not guarantee that she would be able to marry a millionaire, but that as far as her nasal appearance was concerned, that certainly could be addressed. It was decided that she would undergo a standard reduction rhinoplasty, along with a very small chin implant. As her facial features were quite youthful, no other surgery was indicated.

The operation was successful. She had an uncomplicated postoperative course and, after a few months, was "lost to follow-up."

I hadn't heard from her for about three years when I received a Christmas card from her new residence in Montana. It seems that after completing the year in Connecticut, she decided to move back to her hometown in Montana. When she arrived there, she met her high school sweetheart whom she had not seen in over 25 years. He had remained single and, as is so often the case with ranches, inherited his parents' cattle ranch when they passed away. He was now the owner of several thousand acres of land, several thousand cows, and was clearly financially very successful. They rekindled their high school romance, got married, and, to date, are living happily ever after. As she wrote in her Christmas card, "I went home, met my high school sweetheart, and ended up marrying a millionaire."

It turns out that cosmetic surgery can be helpful for some patients in areas other than appearance. Sometimes (though not be counted on), fairy tales do come true.

MY PATIENT, MY COLLEAGUE

HARRY J. BUNCKE, M.D.   SAN MATEO, CA

What does not destroy me,
makes me stronger.
–Nietzsche

Dr. Franco was a plastic surgery resident in the general hospital in Mexico, where Fernando Montastereo, who was well known to all American plastic surgeons, was chief. During the terrible earthquake of 1985, the resident and intern quarters, which were next to the hospital, crumbled like a deck of cards. Nine stories just fell. Dr. Franco and his roommate were on the fourth floor. His roommate was killed. Dr. Franco survived, but his hand was trapped. All four fingers were crushed under tons of cement, and he couldn't move.

Approximately 30-40 residents and fellows were killed during the quake. The search for survivors went on for days. Fortunately, Dr. Franco had seven brothers who looked night and day, crawling through the rubble trying to find him. Finally, one of his brothers heard him yelling. They dug him out. Dr. Franco's fingers were gangrenous and crushed beyond salvage. One of the residents who had trained in a microsurgical laboratory attempted to revascularize the fingers. But it turned out the fingers were not viable, and they had to amputate all four fingers just distal to the metacarpal phalangeal joints.

In order to preserve length, they placed Dr. Franco's hand in a traditional groin flap. Well, this took months to heal, as he had to also deal with infections. Finally, after a year, Fernando

Montastereo arranged to have him transferred to our hospital in San Francisco, where we put a team together and did a double microvascular transplant of the second toe from the right foot and the left foot to the ring and little finger positions. This allowed the fingers to grip things against the thumb. Fortunately, Dr. Franco's thumb was in good shape. But the proximal palm was badly crushed so we had to use another microvascular flap. In all, we really performed three microvascular transplants. Two at one sitting and the third at another sitting. In a period of two years, Dr. Franco came to our hospital several times. He actually trained and did microsurgical techniques in the lab to develop his dexterity. With dedication and effort, he went back and joined the residency program. He finished his residency in plastic surgery and is now practicing plastic surgery in Tijuana, Mexico. What a joy it is to see a patient become a colleague.

He married a lovely American girl whom we all met, and they have two children. Several members of the staff that operated on him, as well as the hand therapist, went to his wedding in Mexico City. It was quite an occasion. It was one of the few parties that I have gone to that I had to leave to go and sleep while the others continued to drink, dance, and sing well past 5 o'clock in the morning.

I, TOO, CAN SUE

SAMUEL ROSENTHAL, M.D.
JACKSONVILLE, FL

Idealism is what precedes experience;
cynicism is what follows.
  –David T. Wolf

This relates to a patient, a 45-year-old lady who, in 1978, two years after having undergone intestinal bypass surgery for morbid obesity, requested a tummy tuck for marked redundancy of skin and weakness of the abdominal wall. She had lost over 100 pounds following that intestinal bypass which was performed just about in that period of time. She, unfortunately, developed an ileus after surgery, but otherwise her recovery was uncomplicated.

Approximately, one year later, after an additional moderate weight loss of about 10-20 pounds, the patient was offered a revision as a courtesy at no charge. The patient was admitted the night before surgery and at that time we found that her potassium was low. Because of her previous ileus problem, we elected to discharge her and have her get her potassium in order. Subsequently, she filed suit.

I had an attorney who knew her call to find out why on earth she had filed suit. He basically stated, "After 20 minutes of conversation with Mrs. X, she felt that you no longer loved her." (i.e., I did not give her an appointment to see me; I simply said, "When your potassium is normal, make an appointment." But I did not specify when and so forth.) Whatever the reason, she did indeed file suit, which was subsequently thrown out by the judge in town; I received a summary judgment. Thirty days later, I hired an attorney, advising him that I wanted no funds from this case, and filed a counter suit for malicious prosecution against both attorney and patient. This was well received by the local media, and I won the case.

Ironically, this surgery was one of the best results I have ever achieved in abdominoplasty in terms of contrast (the woman had a barrel belly). In addition, I made house calls on this lady as she lived 10 minutes from my home. It simply illustrates that no matter what rapport you have established with a patient, one never knows when one is going to be sued.

Chapter VII
Humorous

BACK-TO-FRONT

BARRY ZIDE, M.D.   NEW YORK, NY

> *More drown in puddles than in the sea.*
> —Russian proverb

New York University Medical Center was where I carried out a routine breast reduction procedure. My assistant was one of the newer residents, a young man about thirty-three years old who had been married for three or four years. He was stable, steady, and competent; in every way, he was an excellent surgeon.

The operation was completed without difficulty. I taped the wounds and asked the resident to place the postoperative bra, a garment which hooked together at the front. I left the operating room and went back to my office, satisfied that the patient and her healing process would be in good shape.

It was with some surprise that I received an urgent call the next morning from my patient, "Dr. Zide, I'm in incredible pain. You have to see me immediately!" My mind raced quickly over the possibilities . . . a hematoma, perhaps? . . . or a blood clot? . . . some kind of problem with a nerve? I would have to examine her, so I asked her to come in as soon as possible.

Within a few minutes she arrived. I helped her to undress and was dumbfounded to see that the strap of the bra was directly across the center of her breasts, and the cups at the back! All I had to do was gently reverse the garment so the cups were supporting the breasts as they were designed to do, and the lady's pain immediately subsided.

She thanked me effusively, much relieved to know that nothing serious was involved with her discomfort. Then, as soon as she left, I paged the resident who had assisted me. He quickly called back. "Do me a favor," I said. "Tell me what you were thinking when you put that postoperative bra on our patient. The cups were in the back, and I just don't get it."

His reply was simple. "Well," he said, "My wife's bra hooks in the back. It never occurred to me that they made them any other way!"

PARTING SHOT

BARRY ZIDE, M.D.   **NEW YORK, NY**

A joke is an epitaph for an emotion.
–Nietzsche

Seventy-two-year-old Sonya suffered from a gross disfigurement of her face. The cause was a vascular malformation of her upper lip which made her appearance so grotesque that she would not allow it to be seen by anybody. To add to her lonely agony, the condition involved constant bleeding.

The effect of this situation was that she had been in self-imposed isolation for five years. The only occasions upon which she would leave the house (which had become her prison) were to buy food and, while on these infrequent expeditions, she invariably wore a mask.

She had four children, but they became so harassed by their mother's increasing neurosis, so disturbed by her frequent telephone calls to say that she was bleeding to death, that they all eventually left New York City. The constant running to and fro, catering to her extreme anxiety, reached a point where it was just too much for them.

Her life receded to a single point of psychological pain. Not surprisingly, she became totally unable to cope with life. After so many years of loneliness (her husband had died twenty years earlier), she was, quite literally, a recluse.

At last, recognizing the hopelessness of her position, she

came to me for help. A glimmer of light, of hope, must have cut through the gloom of her existence to bring her to an understanding that plastic surgery could possibly provide relief from her misery. I cut out the entire malformation except for an outcrop inside the cheek. Being post-menopausal meant that the problem did not continue to grow. The procedure changed her appearance from grotesque to virtually normal, and the bleeding stopped, as did her anxiety about that factor.

Another element now came into the situation. She became pathologically dependent on me, so I saw her every week for three or four months. She unburdened herself by telling me that for the first time in ten years she had gone away on a trip, that she planned to visit her grandchildren in Washington, D.C., and that she no longer needed to wear her mask when she went out.

We reached the stage when she was able to accept that we could now terminate the weekly visits and that her transformation was complete. Seventy-two-year-old Sonya came into my office for the last time and laid down on the operating table, as she had so often before. I checked for some slight pulsations in her cheek and decided that some final words of encouragement were in order. "Sonya," I said, "You've had a tough time for the last fifteen or twenty years. You've had trouble with your family, you've lived a lonely life, but now it's time for you to go out and do stuff for yourself. Is there anything you really want for yourself now that this thing's pretty much straightened out?"

You know, a surgeon's life prepares one for the unexpected and brings answers to questions fairly rapidly, as events can move quickly when dealing with the human body, but for the only time in my life that I can remember, I was truly lost for words when she replied. She looked at me with a completely straight face and said, "An orgasm wouldn't hurt." I mean, what do you say to that?

FREE FALL

JAMES W. MAY, JR., M.D. BOSTON, MA

Perched on the loftiest throne in the world,
we are still sitting on our own behind.
—Montaigne

Some twenty years ago I took on the responsibility of organizing a session of an American Association for Hand Surgery program. The session was entitled "A Night on Emergency Hand Call," and consisted of a group of four invited panelists, with myself as moderator, who would be presented with difficult hand patient problems about which to opine and suggest treatment. This method of presentation allowed members of the audience to see panelists being put on the spot, just the same as they themselves would be when seeing a patient on Emergency Hand Call in the local community.

The surgeons who comprised the panel were to be seated on a raised platform, three feet above floor level, where they could be easily seen by the audience. Their discussions about the various cases presented would be augmented by slide presentations on a screen visible to both themselves and the viewers.

It was my privilege to have Dr. Lynn Puckett, Chairman of Plastic Surgery at the University of Missouri, accept my invitation to be on the panel. He is not only an expert in hand surgery but very gifted in verbalizing his opinions and treatment plan for audience consideration.

Dr. Puckett was slightly late in arriving for the panel. When

212

he entered to join the seated group, the lights had been dimmed during the initial case presentation to allow for projected slides to be easily viewed. As a result, he was forced to take the chair closest to the screen and farthest from the moderator, as all the remaining chairs had been taken by the other panelists.

The time arrived for Lynn to comment on a case which was being presented orally and by a selection of slides on the screen. His angle of vision was such that he needed to reposition his chair farther back so that he could clearly see the screen. It was unfortunate that this move took the back legs of his chair over the edge of the elevated platform. He executed a near acrobatic back-flip, head over heels, onto the floor three feet below.

The audience registered two memorable components of the episode. First was the ungraceful nature of his disappearance from the panel. The second, and more impressive, was caused by his having the microphone staying attached to his tie. The expletive uttered by Dr. Puckett during the free-fall component of his exodus, broadcast loudly to the entire audience, will be forever remembered in the annals of hand surgery.

With great good fortune, the only injury was to Dr. Puckett's ego.

BIMBO!

JUAN CARLOS GIACHINO, M.D.
STUART, FL

When choosing between two evils, I always like to
try the one I've never tried before.
–Mae West

The setting for this little vignette was the operating room of a local hospital.

The cast of characters:

The patient – A seventy-five-year-old man who was being treated under straight local anesthesia for the excision of multiple skin lesions on various areas of his body;

The surgeon (that's me) – Trained in Argentina and America, my native language is Spanish, but I am fluent in English, although heavily accented, and have a broad com-mand of vocabulary;

The scrub nurse – A nurse who worked privately for me;

The staff nurse – Assigned to circulate and monitor the patient, a good-looking lady in her mid-thirties.

Let the scrub nurse take up the tale . . .

"We placed our patient in the supine position on the OR table, then marked, injected, and excised all the lesions on the anterior surfaces of his body. The patient tolerated this well, so the surgeon planned to continue by excising as many of the lesions on his back as possible.

"To achieve this, the patient had to be turned and repositioned. He would need to roll over onto his side and settle into a comfortable position so that I could re-prep and re-drape him. Dr. G directed him to turn, and the patient, wanting to make sure he did exactly as his doctor required, asked which way he should go.

"The doctor tried to be as explicit as possible, saying, 'Turn over onto your right side so you're facing the blonde bimbo sitting beside you.' Hearing this, the cute little old man chuckled as he turned to his right.

"Linda, the staff nurse, and I looked over the tops of our masks at each other as if to say 'Did you hear what I think I heard?' Having been Dr. G's private scrub for several years, I knew him well enough to know that he didn't have the foggiest notion of what he'd just said, or how insulting he sounded. His demeanor was not that of someone who had just made a joke.

"I glanced at Linda again and could tell that whatever she was thinking, it wasn't good. While being as diplomatic with the doctor as I could, I quietly asked him if he thought it was a good idea to insult our circulator. His obvious bafflement immediately confirmed my suspicion that he didn't know what he'd just said. I asked him what he thought the word 'bimbo' meant, and he replied that he thought it meant 'a beautiful, blonde girl.'

"We held an emergency vocabulary lesson in American slang. Dr. G immediately broke scrub and went over to apologize and hug the 'bimbo.'

"During this interlude, Linda extracted a promise of free future cosmetic surgery!"

STUTTER

JUAN CARLOS GIACHINO, M.D.
STUART, FL

Take care and say this with presence of mind.
—Terence

The scene was my office operating room where the patient was having a breast procedure under local anesthesia with intravenous conscious sedation.

I was carrying out the operation, assisted by my private scrub nurse and my circulating nurse. The circulator, a highly experienced and competent RN, had the handicap of a speech impediment, a severe stutter.

The case was going ahead with the patient sedated, prepped, and draped. The circulator was monitoring the patient from the other side of the ether screen and filling out the operative record. She wanted to be sure that the form was completed correctly, so she confirmed the pre-op diagnosis by reading it out loud.

"Dr Giachino, the p-p-p-patient die-die-die-die . . ."

A <u>long</u> pause followed.

I stepped back from the table. I felt every sphincter in my body tighten, and I was sure that I was having a heart attack . . . until I saw the monitor screens giving their signals of life.

Finally, the circulating nurse got out her complete interrogative: "Dr. Giachino, the p-p-patient's d-d-diagnosis, p-p-please?"

216

TIME WARP

KELMAN I. COHEN, M.D.   RICHMOND, VA

Life is the art of drawing sufficient conclusions
from insufficient premises.
–Samuel Butler

Together with a colleague, I had been in practice at the Medical College of Virginia for about a year. Neither of us had yet seen an aesthetic case until one day when a fifty-something lady, Mrs. Jones, came into my office to express interest in a facelift.

I discovered that Dr. Ken Pickerell of Duke University had recommended me as a young and talented plastic surgeon. It was not Mrs. Jones' first encounter with aesthetic surgery; Dr. Pickerell had performed a rhinoplasty for her several years earlier.

My patient-to-be was an unusual character. Her accent was outlandish, and you could be forgiven if you took her voice as that of a comedian mimicking some grande dame from high society. She was rich as Croesus and led a lavish existence in her castle-like Richmond home.

Memorable? Oh, she was memorable, all right . . .

We decided to go ahead with the operation she had requested. Back in those days, a facelift was an inpatient procedure. Our plastic surgery facility was a twelve-bed ward of tiny rooms which had been converted from the Pediatrics Department. The nursing staff had never taken care of a cosmetic patient before – most of our beds were occupied by people with gunshot wounds, facial fractures, and hand and spinal cord injuries. So, Dr. Dawson, my colleague, and I spent a lot of time orienting the nurses to the needs and challenges of the aesthetic patient. We even went so far as to have some cosmetic work done on the room itself to more pleasantly accommodate our wealthy uptown guest.

Surgery went well. The next morning, Dawson and I walked into her room to find her sitting up in bed and looking rather perky. We were relieved to see that the facial nerve moved and that there was no hematoma.

"How was last night – not too bad, I hope – after surgery?" I asked her.

"Rather pleasant and somewhat amusing," she smilingly replied.

"Why was that?," I queried. It was not the sort of comment we usually heard from a postoperative patient.

"Well," she said, "about two o'clock in the morning the lights were switched on, and I was awakened by two teenagers. One of them asked, 'Where's Effie Jones?' I told them, 'I'm afraid you have the wrong Mrs. Jones.' 'Oh,' they both replied. They didn't leave at once and, after a few seconds, the other one asked, 'Lady, why are you all wrapped up in that big bandage?' "

My patient chuckled at the memory of the conversation, then went on.

"I told them that the bandage was there because I had a facelift. 'A facelift? What's that?' they wanted to know, so I explained that a facelift is an operation that makes you younger. 'My God, Lady,' they replied. 'How old are you today, and how old were you yesterday?' "

MIXED SIGNALS

PETER NEUMANN, M.D.   GREAT NECK, NY

> *Do not remove a fly from your friend's head*
> *with a hatchet.*
> –Chinese Proverb

In my first year as a plastic surgery resident I ran into a situation which combined in equal parts black humor and harsh drama.

I was acting as second assistant on a breast reduction operation carried out by Doctor Bromberg, Chief of the Department of Plastics. He followed his customary procedure – a free nipple graft for a very large breast reduction.

His routine was to take off the right nipple, put it in a gauze, and hand it to the nurse. Then off with the left nipple. The nurse took care of both nipples, their gauzes marked L and R, and placed them on the back part of the operating table.

The surgeon continued his work, and then Chance dealt an unfair hand. As the operation went on, the nurses changed. It so happened that it was the relief nurse's first time in the operating room – she had joined the staff from nursing school only two weeks before.

She came to the table thoroughly imbued with the lessons in tidiness and hygiene that had been emphasized by her nursing education. Unseen by the doctors who were, of course, focused entirely on their work, she took the two gauzes containing the nipples and threw them into the wastebasket.

We finished shaping the breasts, and the chief asked for the right nipple.

The phrase "my blood ran cold" might be an overused one, but that is exactly what happened to me when I looked toward the back table and saw no gauze pads there. I spun around to the nurse.

"What happened to the two gauze pads that were in the back?"

"Well, when I came in an hour ago, I cleaned up."

"You <u>cleaned up</u>?" I repeated foolishly. There seemed nothing else to say.

The chief had heard this brief exchange. He looked hard at me.

"Neumann, it's either your nipples or the patient's nipples. You have three minutes to find them."

My already chilled bloodstream became a cold sweat when I heard his words – I knew he was not kidding. I spun around and began going through the garbage, as well as the sponges that had been discarded from the table. By doing this, I knew that I was breaking the stringent sterile conditions required of an OR doctor or nurse, and that I would have to scrub up again before returning to the table.

Five unsuccessful minutes later, I gulped and confessed to the chief that I couldn't find them.

He did not reply to me, but turned to the new nurse (her first day, remember!) and said "Dear, take off your shirt. We're removing your nipples." Her face contorted in fear, she screamed an ear-piercing scream, and ran headlong out of the operating room. Even after she had gone we heard her crying in the distance.

The head nurse came into the OR and reprimanded the doctor, as was only to be expected. But luck came to the rescue. When she entered the room I found the nipples wrapped up in their gauze packages in the bottom of one of the throwaway baskets. A new scrub nurse came into the room and finished the case with us.

The patient never turned a hair. Both nipples subsequently healed with no problems.

CEDAR CHOPPERS

T. WILKINSON, M.D.   SAN ANTONIO, TX

Hope springs eternal in the human breast;
Man never is, but always to be blest.
    —Alexander Pope

The cedar choppers of south Texas come very close to being true nomadic hillbillies. Itinerant souls, they travel from ranch to ranch, living under primitive and uncivilized conditions. They make their meager living by clearing the cedar trees that suck the goodness out of the soil of south Texas ranches.

The only time they can be seen in town is when they bring their logs in for sale. They are a most unusual group. Inbred, too, if truth be told.

My office in the town's medical center is tasteful, unobtrusive, and discreet. My patients normally fit the same low-key pattern, and so it was with some surprise that I encountered a large, muscular cedar chopper arriving for an appointment.

"Hello," I said, I'm Dr. Wilkinson. How can I help you?"

"Doc," said the burly man, "I need me some titties."

I tried with some difficulty to preserve my professional demeanor.

"I see. And you can let me have a reason for this need of yours?"

222

"Yeah." His voice was gruff, a rural *basso profundo.* "I want to be a woman."

I swallowed hard. "OK." I went on to explain: "Well, you'll have to get used to the idea of wearing a dress, you'll need to act like a woman, and of course hormone therapy will be required." I was beginning to sweat just a little, and I hoped that my voice did not betray my nervousness. "Eventually I'm sure that you will need to have the sex-change operation."

"Naw, Doc, I don't want none of that. I just want me some titties so the boys in the bunkhouse will have something to play with!"

I told you that they are unusual people.

IMMUNITY TO AGE

WILLIAM H. FRAZIER, M.D.
VERO BEACH, FL

There is no cure for birth and death
save to enjoy the interval.
–Santayana

It's all of twenty years since I first met Mrs. Pamela Lawrence. She was a lady in her early seventies, well dressed and adorned with expensive jewelry, and with impeccable manners. In conversation with her, I found that she was originally from Germany, lived at very much a "right" address, and that she and her husband fell clearly into the multimillionaire category. Among other assets, they owned large land holdings in Michigan. She told me about her daughter, who was in her mid-fifties at that time, and about her son-in-law.

Mrs. Lawrence (even today, I would think of it as an impertinence to call her "Pamela") came to me to discuss the possibilities of facial rejuvenation. She'd had a facelift some ten years before, but she felt that her appearance was beginning to show the signs of age.

We agreed that surgery would be appropriate for her. I carried out a face-lift with special attention to the upper and lower eyelids, and the result was extremely pleasing. Her husband was so taken with her youthfully renewed features that he immediately planned a grand party for her – fifty or so guests, haute cuisine catering, bar, the whole works – just three days after surgery! I was able to persuade him that it

224

was a bit too soon after the procedure, and he grudgingly postponed the event for another five days.

When the celebration actually took place, the guest list had grown to over a hundred. My patient greeted everybody at the door, was cordial and sociable for more than two hours, and then retired to her bedroom, tired but quite obviously very happy.

A dark shadow fell across her life only six months later, when her husband of so many years died. As a new widow, she nevertheless continued her life of great propriety in demeanor, dress, and adornment. But after ten years of single status, she once again felt that she was beginning to show signs of aging, and didn't like that at all.

Mrs. Lawrence decided that a third facelift would be desirable, and again came to me for consultation. I agreed with her. Once more, the procedure was uneventful and successful. She felt that this repeat renewal of her youthful appearance was much more consistent with her optimistic mental outlook and her many and various social activities.

She focused on the enjoyment of different places. Each year she traveled to Europe, in the company of her daughter and son-in-law. Summers were spent in her home state of Michigan, winters in the relaxed warmth of Florida. A truly enviable lifestyle.

Still the urge to retain the sparkle of her youth was alive in her. Six months before reaching the age of ninety, in October, she felt that what she called "touch-up work" would be in order, to get her in fine shape for her birthday. Once more, she asked for my services in performing a fourth facelift. And once more, the operation went without incident, and once more the result was highly beneficial. Her appearance was now that of a woman perhaps twenty or thirty years younger than her ninety years.

During the many years that I had known Mrs. Lawrence, she and my wife had met socially and became good friends. A month after the last surgery, the two of them made arrangements to visit Germany, where my patient could spend two weeks on a nostalgic return visit. Here she renewed ties with all her family who were still alive, and with old friends. They visited the Berlin homestead where she had been born, the hotels where she and her husband had stayed, and many other places associated with her younger days.

The most interesting thing for me, however, was that during their travels, my fifty-four-year-old wife and her much older friend were taken to be sisters; they both had dark hair and fairly similar features. Clearly, people could tell that my patient was the older of the two, but some confusion was always evident from their daily cocktail ritual.

Promptly at five o'clock every afternoon, they ordered drinks – a large vodka on the rocks and a glass of white wine. Invariably, the waiter would place the wine in front of Mrs. Lawrence and the hard liquor in front of my wife. Just as invariably, they would exchange glasses and then laugh about the waiter's assumption that the wine should be for the senior member of the pair.

After they returned to the States, my patient continued with her idyllic life. A further twist in the relationship issue now became evident. She began to go out fairly regularly with her daughter and her son-in-law. When the three met people who did not known them, again the assumption was that the two women were sisters. The extra misconception was that the son-in-law was Mrs. Lawrence's husband and that the daughter was single.

* * * * * * * * * *

As I write, my patient is ninety-two-years old, still travels north and south within the U.S. each year, still takes an occasional trip to Europe, still drinks her two vodka on the rocks (one at five, the other at dinner), and still smokes every afternoon and evening. She recently confided in me that her biggest concern is that she is putting on weight. She actually turns the scale at about a hundred and ten pounds and has put on perhaps two pounds in the last twenty years; but she feels that her size 4 clothes don't look as well on her now as they used to.

Is liposuction in this ninety-two year old's future? Probably not, but it's certainly gratifying, even exciting, to find someone like Pamela Lawrence, who seems to be immune to the aging process, even while growing older gracefully and inspiring her doctor.

Who knows – she may need a fifth facelift before her hundredth birthday!

MORE IS BETTER

GARRY S. BRODY, M.D.   LOS ANGELES, CA

Nothing succeeds like excess.
–Wilde

I was referred a 27-year-old young woman (by her gynecologist) for a facelift. I knew this gynecologist well, and I'm sure that the referral was primarily for me to give her the "grandfatherly talk." It turns out she was an exotic dancer; and her agent had recommended she get a facelift so as to be more attractive.

In the course of my long discourse at discouraging her, it was apparent that she was holding up very heavy breasts with her folded forearms and I could not resist commenting on how uncomfortable she seemed. She stated, "Yes, they're terribly uncomfortable. I had 1000-cc implants placed." On further questioning, it turns out that she was a D-cup before the augmentation and these were inserted by an east-coast Chairman of Plastic Surgery. She states that she had only wanted 500-cc implants, but that her agent had talked the doctor into placing 1000-cc implants while she was asleep.

I examined her and, indeed, she did have a remarkable bosom. I began to suggest to her ways in which we could lighten her burden when she interrupted me by saying, "Doctor, what you don't understand is that since I've had these implants, my income has gone up $2000 a week!"

228

A MATTER OF ORDER

GARRY S. BRODY, M.D.   LOS ANGELES, CA

I have an instinct for loving the truth;
but only an instinct.
–Voltaire

This patient was an African-American with a fractured jaw whom I cared for during my residency. In those days, there was a lot of closed reduction and fixation, and hospital stays were much longer than today. Every morning as I made rounds, I would put my fingers in his mouth to feel if the wires were tight or rubbing, and then I would wash my hands to go on to the next patient.

One day, the patient said to me, "Doc, you're supposed to wash your hands *before* you put them in my mouth, not *after*."

FEEL LIKE A NEW MAN

HILTON BECKER, M.D.   BOCA RATON, FL

Tact consists of knowing how far to go in going too far.
—Cocteau

A patient with very large breasts, one might say extremely large breasts, inquired as to how she would feel after the breast reduction surgery. With that, the attending surgeon looked up at her and said,

"After your breast reduction, my dear, you'll feel like a new <u>man</u>."

DROP DEAD GORGEOUS

JOHN CHURCH, M.D.   NEW ORLEANS, LA

Men who pass most comfortably through the world
are those who possess good digestions and hard hearts.
–Harriet Martineau

When I was a resident, I had a rotation at the public health hospital. We could do cosmetic surgery there and let our patients kind of hide while they recovered because there was no urgency in discharging them from the hospital.

I did my first forehead lift on a lady in mid-December sometime. Of course, she got the world's biggest hematoma. I drained it, and it still looked kind of a mess. Finally, it got to be Christmas; she wondered if she could go see her brother who was in town. She hadn't seen him in a number of years. I consented to let her out on a pass, even though she was not quite ready for the public.

When she returned, she was in tears. I asked her what happened, as I thought she'd be pleased to see her brother. She said that while she was happy to see him, he took one look at her, had a heart attack, and died on the spot.

So, now I have to list in my Informed Consent, "Death of a relative," I suppose.

EYE OF THE BEHOLDER

MAXWELL A. COOPER, M.D.
KAILUA, HI

*It is a law of nature that we defend ourselves from one
affectation only by means of another.*
–Valeny

When I was a very young plastic surgeon at a military teaching hospital, I was approached by a patient of mine for whom I had done a considerable amount of reconstructive surgery with a request for "a dimple."

I told her that she was in great luck because I had just read in our national journal a paper on how to make facial dimples.

I said, "You meant dimples, of course." She advised me that no, she only wished one dimple on the right cheek.

I performed this procedure and the result was very satisfactory. She told me some months later of her experience when her husband and she took an old friend to the club for drinks. After a few, he leaned across at her and said in slurred speech, "Louise, I have always admired your dimple."

She felt that was the ultimate compliment to herself and to my efforts.

THE BEST MEDICINE

PAUL R. WEISS, M.D. NEW YORK, NY

A joke is an epitaph on an emotion.
–Nietzsche

As well as being a fine doctor, Bruce Bendel was the most accomplished mimic I ever met. His powers of impersonation were legendary. Together with his innate sense of humor, he could have chosen a career in entertainment as readily as one in medicine.

I came across Bendel in the spring of 1972. I was in the last month of my second year in general surgery residency at Montefiore Medical Center in New York's Bronx and expected an important rotation on the plastic surgery service at Montefiore. Being greatly interested in securing a plastic surgery residency, I was eager to impress the Department Chairman, Michael Lewin.

Bruce Bendel was the plastic surgery service's chief resident at that time. Legend has it that he deployed his talent for imitation by convincing callers that his telephone voice was that of Dr. Lewin himself, with hilarious, but sometimes disconcerting, results.

Dr. Lewin's stern approach to plastic surgery training, especially in the operating room, was in vivid contrast to Bendel's ability to find humor in any and every situation. On many occasions while we were awaiting Dr. Lewin's arrival in the OR, Bruce would launch into one of his superb

"Lewin take-offs." With amazing accuracy, he would mimic every subtle nuance of the Department Chairman's mien, European-accented speech, and behavior. The self-control of everyone in the OR would be severely challenged when the real Dr. Lewin entered the room, speaking and acting normally but precisely in the manner which Bendel had so cleverly imitated.

My last day on the service followed the usual pattern. Dr. Bendel and I prepared a patient for surgery in the operating room – multiple burn scar revisions which were to be done under local anesthesia. Throughout the preparation routine, Bendel continued his humorous Lewin impersonation which kept me laughing.

Finally, the OR was prepared, the patient was on the table, and Dr. Lewin entered. I had barely regained my composure when Dr. Lewin addressed me personally in exactly the same voice, intonation, and accent that Bendel had been imitating just seconds earlier.

The controlled levity of the situation was made more complex by another factor. Bendel was highly regarded as a plastic surgery resident, but in the eyes of his chief, he could do nothing right and was the target of constant criticism from Dr. Lewin (a situation not, I might add, unknown to residents everywhere). Suddenly, the amplified voice of a surgical resident blared into the OR over the intercom. The atmosphere, tense with suppressed laughter, reinforced the perceived shortcomings of Bendel, and made Dr. Lewin give vent to his detestation of intercom interruptions of surgical procedures.

"DON'T USE IT!" he shouted at the loudspeaker.

The loud, gruff voice, heavy with his European accent, echoed Bendel's faultless portrayal. I almost shook with silent laughter, but somehow we managed to complete the case. Dr. Lewin prepared to leave, giving instructions for patient care, for skin closure, and for dressings.

The scene as the door closed behind Dr. Lewin that day was unimaginable. Bendel and I burst out laughing. The patient – draped so she could not see the surgery team, and thus unaware of Dr. Lewin's exit – not unnaturally asked about the laughter.

Bendel replied in perfect mimicry of his chief, "Be quiet and cooperate." Needless to say, this final jab dispelled what composure I had left, but Dr. Lewin's orders were carried out, and we left the operating room.

I don't know if the patient ever asked Dr. Lewin, himself, about these events and the hilarity in the OR that day, but I am certain that he must have found out what had transpired. It could not have been otherwise.

AUTHOR'S NOTE:

Tragically, within weeks of completing his plastic surgery residency that June, Dr. Bruce Bendel was diagnosed with leukemia. He died a short time later – much too early in life, and long before he had a chance to make his mark and reputation in plastic surgery.

IF IT'S IN PRINT, IT MUST BE TRUE

ROBERT M. GOLDWYN, M.D.
BROOKLINE, MA

Perched on the loftiest throne in the world,
we are still sitting on our own behind.
–Montaigne

My first few years in practice may have lacked money, but not comedy. I remember well an incident that involved an elderly male whom I saw because of a skin cancer on his face. He had a lesion that merited excision. At the time of the operation, he told me that I had really impressed him.

"You are so young to be so successful. You must have a lot of energy, going back and forth between Boston and Miami," he said.

"What do you mean?," I asked, since I had not been to Miami for at least five years.

"Well, you have an office in Miami," he replied, looking confused.

"I do?" I replied.

"Well, that's what your card says," he informed me, and showed me a card that my secretary had given him. In fact, he was partially correct.

A printing error had my name with a Miami address. Somehow, at the printer, my cards and those of another surgeon had become joined. By throwing away a few other misprinted cards, I closed my Miami office!

TOUGH LOVE

ROBERT N. COOPER, M.D.   STUART, FL

Sentimental irony is a dog that bays at the moon
while he pisses on a grave.
–Kierkegaard

A little over six years ago, before we moved to our new surgery center, I did a facelift for an absolutely delightful fellow. At that time, my office was on the same body of water it is now. Adjoining that surgery center was an annex that had multiple apartments. A distinguished-looking gentleman with classic good looks had checked into one of the apartments. His long-term partner of some thirty years had accompanied him to the consultation and then to the threshold of surgery.

My patient was in his late-60s and his partner, a former entertainer, was in his mid-50s. Over the next six years, these two fellows became real friends of the practice and me, personally. As long as I've been in practice, I've spent three weeks of the month in Florida, operating, and seeing patients, and the fourth week in New York seeing preoperative consultations and postoperative follow-up patients. While in New York, the nurses, staff, and my personal ladyfriend all go out together and, on more than once occasion, we've hooked up with Allen and Jeffrey. They're witty, charming, and just plain fun, and yet this delightful couple generated one of the cruelest stories I can relate from my practice.

Confident that his partner, Allen, was in good hands, Jeffrey decided to go out and get his nails done. Jeffrey is a flamboyant character and quite gregarious. He came to the office that day wearing glasses with a bright red plastic frame and a matching red-framed Japanese fan. Our receptionist was delighted to refer him to a nail salon within easy walking distance of the office. Jeffrey announced that he would be back after his manicure to see how Allen was doing.

Allen's surgery went quite well. He was brought back to the apartment and I made a housecall there early that evening. It was certainly not unusual to see Jeffrey sitting at the foot of Allen's bed, fanning himself, looking at Allen. As I came into the room, Allen, now several hours post-discharge from the surgery center was waking up from a nap. He still had some of the effects of sedation in his system and clearly was not completely lucid. Innocently, he called out, "Mommy, Mommy, I want my Mommy." Jeffrey, seated at the foot of the bed, fanning himself nonchalantly, looked lovingly at his partner and said rather assertively, "Oh, shutup, you don't have a mother. You're an orphan."

I almost fell backwards in shock. I could not help but laugh. It was probably the cruelest thing I had ever heard anyone say to a patient waking up from sedation. It was also one of the funniest things I ever heard. On multiple occasions since that time, over a dinner table at their home or at my home, we've laughed about that same story together.

DON'T JUDGE A BOOK BY ITS COVER

STANLEY TAUB, M.D.   NEW YORK, NY

No man is exempt from saying silly things;
the mischief is to say them deliberately.
–Montaigne

A mother brought her daughter in for a rhinoplasty consultation. The young lady was 19 years old and had a nasal hump deformity. Her mother quietly listened during the consultation as I explained the procedure and demonstrated how I could improve her daughter's nose.

After I finished the consultation, I asked if they had any questions. The mother stared at my nose and asked, "How come the tailor doesn't wear good clothes?"

VIVA LAS VEGAS

T. WILKINSON, M.D.   SAN ANTONIO, TX

The two things that a healthy person hates most between heaven and hell are a woman who is not dignified and a man who is.
–Chesterton

During one of our seminars we were demonstrating how to accelerate the recovery from liposuction with a new external ultrasound called XUAL.

One of the patients that I had planned to do in the seminar was a Las Vegas showgirl and a star in her own right. She agreed to come down a week or two early to have her breast implant replacement and external ultrasound to shrink the wrinkling in her abdomen. She really didn't need an abdominoplasty and had almost no body fat, but I wanted to show that we had tightened her considerably. During the seminar, she agreed to have anesthetic placed in the area and let us demonstrate once more how to do this for technique.

So, she's stretched out in the exam room with a dozen or so doctors and nurses gathered around, and we proceeded to demonstrate how the external ultrasound was applied. One of the doctors leaned over to her and said, "You know, you're awfully nice to let people see us doing this."

She replied, "Honey, this is the fewest people who have ever seen me naked in ten years."

240

Chapter VIII
The Human Condition

A FAREWELL TO ARMS

FREDERICK LUKASH, M.D.
MANHASSET, NY

That he is mad, 'tis true:' 'tis pity; and pity 'tis true.
—Shakespeare

Anthony was a young man from a small Massachusetts milling town who appeared in the emergency room at the Massachusetts General Hospital with both arms having been amputated just above the wrists. Needless to say, this was quite a sight and stirred all the emotions of the emergency room and surgical staff. Anthony was quite lucid in the emergency room and related to the staff that he had experienced a vision which clearly stated, at least in his mind, that if he amputated both of his hands the hostages would be freed from Iran. This was, in fact, 1980; we were in the final months of the Carter administration, where hostage negotiations and rescue attempts had all come to a halt.

Needless to say, Anthony was taken to the operating room with two very aggressive surgical teams working nonstop for 12 hours to reattach Anthony's limbs. Anthony received more attention than he probably had through his combined previous days on earth and, ultimately, left the Massachusetts General Hospital with reasonably functioning hands. He was remanded to treatment at Massachusetts Mental Hospital.

Sometime later, Anthony was released from Mass Mental with a "clean bill of health." He promptly drove to Jamaica Pond and drowned himself.

This is probably an excellent example of "micro" surgery and missing the "macro" picture.

ORPHANED

ABDEL RAOUF ISMAIL, M.D.
DHAHRAN, SAUDI ARABIA

. . . thou that listeneth to the sighs of infants . . .
–Thomas de Quincey

Recent events have highlighted that Islam is a religion which calls for devotion to a high and restrictive moral code. Saudi Arabia is the heartland of the Islamic faith. My experience with a badly hurt child surprised me with its implications for just how far that code might be ignored, even here, in Dhahran.

The social worker from a nearby orphanage brought a severely scarred three-year-old boy to our plastic surgery clinic and asked for help in caring for his disfigurement. The story behind this request was a sad one.

The child was illegitimate. When he was born late one evening, the distraught mother put the baby into a bag and left the pathetic package on the steps of a mosque. Unseen and alone overnight, he was discovered at the early-morning prayer time. He was crying pitifully, and his face was covered with blood which had stained the sheet he was wrapped in. The cause of his injury was attributed to the rats which are often to be seen scampering through the streets of Dhahran late in the evening.

The rats had eaten part of the infant's right eyebrow and forehead. He was taken into the orphanage, where he was looked after and his wounds dressed. He survived, and stayed for the next three years. But, of course, although his

injured tissues healed, he was left with substantial distortion of the right upper eyelid. What remained of the eyebrow was displaced sideways, close to the hairline of his forehead.

We corrected the scarring by a method known as 'tissue expansion,' and did some hair transplant to augment the missing section of eyebrow. In time, the child will grow up with a virtually normal appearance.

The surprise I experienced was not caused by the case of this child only. The shock set in when I found out that he was just one of some forty others – all of them illegitimate – cared for in the orphanage. I learned from the social worker that it is a very common occurrence, children being abandoned at birth and left in front of a mosque to be found by police or garbage men and taken to this institution.

Perhaps even more amazing is to recognize that a female could be full-term pregnant and manage to keep her condition hidden from her family.

Plastic surgery was able to restore this one child's face. But it revealed a more widespread problem, that of babies being left to an uncertain fate immediately after having come into this world. A surgical window, if you will, on the ills of society.

WOMEN AND CHILDREN ONLY

ABDEL RAOUF ISMAIL, M.D.
DHAHRAN, SAUDI ARABIA

Untwisting all the chains that tie the hidden
soul of harmony.
–John Milton

A westerner would not recognize a Saudi wedding celebration. Custom dictates that women must be separated from the men during the festivities; they are not allowed to be visible to men while the marriage ceremony is taking place. The origin of the custom lies deep in Arab and Moslem culture, but it is very strictly observed in my country.

Toward the end of July, 1999, such a wedding took place in a nearby town. Some three hundred women and their young children were celebrating the happy event in a vast tent with only two doors, one at either end. None of the celebrants realized what a dangerous situation they were in.

At the height of the festivities, the bride was positioned on a podium. Unknown to her, or indeed to any of the party, the electrical wiring for the air conditioning system was centered underneath that dais. A short circuit, or some other electrical problem occurred, and suddenly there was a fire.

At that time of year, the weather conditions are hot and humid. Typically, the temperature can reach over 100 degrees Fahrenheit, so conditions are conducive to fire. The great marquee was soon engulfed by the flames; it was evidently made of a very flammable material. Within seconds, the interior scene became chaos. Women and children were screaming, running, trying to escape, but with only two doors they were trapped. Within seconds, the merrymaking had become catastrophe.

The first I knew about the calamity was an emergency call I received in the early evening, saying that a massive fire had occurred in the neighboring town. Minutes later, patients started arriving in our hospital by ambulance, private car, or whatever other means of transport were available. Within less than an hour, we had received forty-five burn victims, all of them women and children. There was, of course, not one man in the group.

Some of them were burned over almost all of their body surface area. We could do nothing for these worst cases except to keep them comfortable. Nearly all of them had died by the early hours of the morning.

Those few with relatively minor burns were triaged and sent to other hospitals. Half of all those who were admitted to our hospital had significant, full thickness burns to 60 per cent of their body surface area.

To manage the many major burns, we had to completely convert one entire floor into a burn unit. Our operating room was shut down except for emergencies, and we operated on two or three burns every day for the next few weeks. At the end of this challenging time, we were left with about ten severely burned patients. The rest were transferred to other hospitals in the Kingdom and overseas, including some who were sent for long-term treatment in the Shriners' Hospital in Galveston, Texas.

The bottom line was that more than seventy women and

children died during the first week after the fire. The exact statistics were kept secret by the Minister of Health, but I suspect that the total number of deaths would have been about a hundred.

The whole disastrous episode resembles another disaster in New York City back in the 1920s, the Triangle shirt factory fire. The catastrophic loss of life in both cases could have been prevented by the simple expedient of providing better and more accessible means of egress.

How many times do we have to have our lessons repeated before learning them?

WITCH CRAFT?

JACOB GOLAN, M.D. JERUSALEM, ISRAEL

Xenophanes speaks thus: And no man knows
distinctly anything, and no man ever will.
  –Diagenes Laertius Pyrrho VIII

My oldest patient was a religious woman, very orthodox, eighty-three years old, when she came to my office requesting evaluation for a facelift. Her advanced age and her devotion to her religion were, to put it mildly, unusual in one seeking cosmetic surgery.

At first, I was a little worried – not so much about the technical aspects of such a procedure, more about what her real motivation was. But she was insistent and rational; it was about time, she told me, that she got rid of all these unsightly wrinkles.

I thought long and hard about my decision, but ultimately concluded that I would go ahead, based on her physical fitness and her being quite sure of what she wanted. So, I operated. Everything went well, and she recuperated easily with few and minor problems.

Only a few weeks after the procedure, during one of her follow-up visits to my office, she wanted to confide in me the real reason for her determined request.

"You see, Dr. Golan, I have eight grandchildren. The youngest of them, a boy, didn't want to see me; he said I was a witch! Well, I looked at myself in the mirror, and realized that he was right – I really did look like a witch. I would have done anything to bring this young grandson back to me."

"That's why I came to you. He's not afraid of me anymore – he comes to visit me of his own free will. I am so very thankful to you!"

POINT OF VIEW

ROBERT E. MALLIN, M.D.   SANTA FE, NM

When I was young, patients were afraid of me.
Now that I am old, I am afraid of patients.
    –Johann Peter Frank

David Doe, a 6-month-old African-American boy, was in a house fire. His parents and their friends were having a wild drinking party and somehow the house caught fire. Everyone escaped except for David, who was left in the back room. He was treated in the intensive care unit by myself and the pediatrician. We saved his life. He required numerous, numerous reconstructive procedures over the years. Once, when he was about fifteen, I did a procedure and he developed a stiff neck and tried to sue me for it – so much for gratitude.

But here's the real hanger. My medical assistant, a couple of years after I retired, sent me an article from the Anchorage newspaper, titled "David Doe Accused and Arrested for Murder." He had murdered two people while robbing a convenience store and was set to go to jail. Well, sometimes you save a life that's worthwhile and sometimes you don't.

COMMAND AT SEA

GERALD VERDI, D.D.S., M.D.
LOUISVILLE, KY

We wholly conquer only what we assimilate.

–Gide

During my plastic surgery residency, I was able to get a glimpse of the chairman of the department, Dr. Leonard Rubin and his two partners, Dr. Bert Bromberg and Dr. Dick Waldon, at play through a story that occurred prior to my start in 1971. These three pioneering men had each made substantial contributions to the field of plastic surgery.

Drs. Rubin and Bromberg were particularly tough. Excellence was not optional. All three men were in command of their material. All of their residents over the years learned to respect, fear, admire, and care for these three pioneers of surgical precision and deft execution of surgical techniques and innovation.

One would expect that three such strong and fiercely individualistic professionals enjoyed a uniformity of excellence in all of their endeavors. The three of them, for reasons ill understood to this day, decided to buy a sailboat. Not just any sailboat, but a Japanese-made 10-meter Samurai sailboat. A precision instrument of a sailboat – completely in character with the three captains who would guide it to adventures on the seas with the attention to detail of a surgeon.

The boat was, in fact, quite elegant and well crafted. It was delivered to Hyannis in Massachusetts. Dr. Bromberg was the only one of the three with any experience boating.

However, it was decided that the seafaring trio would take possession of the craft in Hyannis and sail it back to its new home, Port of Manhasset Harbor on Long Island, New York.

Upon arriving in Hyannis, the Samurai Sailboat, Ltd., representatives decided to accompany the three "Old Salts" on the voyage. The boat was not fully sorted out or fitted out. One of the representatives went into town and bought a compass. The compass was not "swung" or corrected. The needle apparently pointed in the general direction of north.

They cast off and got underway shortly thereafter. While approaching Martha's Vineyard, as the sun was setting, the engine overheated and shut down. Not long after that, Dr. Rubin got seasick and went below in search of medication in the forward cabin. Dr. Bromberg was yelling that, under the circumstances, they should drop anchor. However, he was overruled and they pressed on.

Their advance was again stymied with the discovery of a leak in the fuel tank, but this was fixed. But passing Gay Head, Martha's Vineyard, an errant boom lurched across mid ship and struck Dr. Waldon squarely on the back of his head, propelling him to the deck with some force.

Dr. Rubin appeared on deck after hearing the commotion and, running from the forward cabin, announced that he thought they should abandon ship. This became moot as shortly thereafter they ran aground.

Lights were visible in the distance. Clear of head in a crisis, they jumped into the water with plans to swim ashore in the direction of the lights. They rapidly discovered what most able-bodied seamen learn early on: If you run aground you're probably in the very shallow water – not two feet in this case.

They and the Samurai representatives "walked" to a farmhouse, admittedly through waters with a very light "chop," and called the Coast Guard. The Coast Guard, piecing together the harrowing story, determined that in the absence of a life-threatening situation, the best course for the sailing quintet was to return to their hapless vessel for the evening.

At daybreak, a Mr. Kelly came out to salvage the young vessel. Title to the boat was still with the Samurai representatives. They may have reflected on an honorable hari-kari if they lost their boat and flatly refused. The genial Mr. Kelly offered to tow them off the sandbar for $1,000. Dr. Bromberg initially objected to the perceived high seas robbery but acquiesced upon reflection of the alternatives.

They may have been collectively new to sailing but not to life. The three skippers convinced the Samurai representatives to cough up the $1,000 on the strength of the argument surely supported by marine law, that the boat was originally to have been delivered to Manhasset Harbor.

With the transfer of $1,000 to Mr. Kelly, the boat was pulled from the sandbar. They set sail and later that day arrived at their destination – Manhasset Harbor.

I don't know if they ever used the boat again. When I started my residency in plastic surgery in 1971, the story was related to me, not as a "suburban legend," but as the real deal. None of the residents I know were ever invited on the boat.

Fortunately, command at sea was quite different from command in the OR.

Chapter IX
Recognition of a Job Well Done

EMBOUCHURE

BARRY ZIDE, M.D.   NEW YORK, NY

*Whatever you do, you need courage. Whatever course you decide
upon, there is always someone to tell you that you are wrong.
There are always difficulties arising which tempt you to
believe that your critics are right. To map out a course
of action and follow it to an end requires some
of the same courage which a soldier needs.
Peace has its victories, but it takes brave men to win them.*
—Emerson

I don't play a musical instrument. That's why I didn't know
what the word embouchure meant until I came across Chris
Jordan – not his real name, of course.

Chris was twenty-seven years old, a music major going for
his Ph.D at Columbia University. He played trombone in
the college band that he led. He was entranced by music
and spent every moment either playing or studying.

He came to see me about a cyst in his upper lip that had
been followed by dermatologists for two years or so. The cyst
was in the right nasolabial fold – between lip and nose – and
it had been estimated that surgery to excise it would take
twenty minutes.

I opened up the site, and it was immediately obvious that
this was no cyst, but a hard nodule deep in the skin. I
arranged for a biopsy, and the report came back that this
lump was in fact a melanoma, eight millimeters deep. The
implication of this finding was that I would have to do some
resection of the upper lip. Because the melanoma was

lodged in the muscle of the lip, I knew that after such a procedure he would have great difficulty in pursing the lips.

That was when the word embouchure assumed its importance in my mind. It is the ability of the player of a wind instrument to shape the lips in that special way needed to coax sound out of it.

So this new diagnosis was freighted with elements of double jeopardy. The possible negative prognosis for a melanoma of this type and size was the first. The second – and perhaps in Chris's mind, the more critical – was that the operation to remove the growth could put an end to his playing career. Because of these considerations, I asked the young man's parents to accompany him into my office to review and understand just what we were looking at. He decided to have me go ahead with the procedure. After all, without life, there would be no music.

As good luck would have it, the metastatic workup was negative – the cancer had not begun to spread to other parts of his body. I told him that I would get him on the schedule as soon as possible, and asked him and his parents to wait until I'd fixed a date for the operation.

"As soon as possible" became a somewhat questionable term. I had only just come onto the faculty at New York University, so I didn't carry too much weight in scheduling a slot in the operating room, which was running on an incredibly tight timetable. The operation could not be treated as an emergency, because really it wasn't. My only option was to "borrow" OR time from one of the senior surgeons.

There followed forty-five rather stressful minutes of telephone calls to various surgeons, most of whom were booked for cosmetic surgery and not over-enthusiastic about giving up their time to me. At last my efforts succeeded, and I was grudgingly given enough time in the OR on the following Tuesday afternoon to carry out the wide and deep excision of Philip's melanoma and the subsequent flap closure.

I went back into the waiting room, where the Jordans were still sitting patiently.

"Chris," I said, "it's been a bit difficult finding a slot in the operating room – that's what took me so much time, for which I apologize – but we are all set for next Tuesday afternoon."

There was a long silence.

It was broken by Chris. "Dr. Zide, I would really like to go ahead on Tuesday afternoon, but could you possibly postpone it until Wednesday morning?"

I was not in the best frame of mind to be asked for a delay, as forty-five minutes had just gone down the tubes fixing the Tuesday. It was difficult to understand why the young man would want to put it off for just one day.

"Chris, what could possibly be so important to you to want to change Tuesday to Wednesday? We have to get this melanoma off your face, and I've just spent three quarters of an hour pleading with more senior surgeons to let me have the time in the OR. And now you want to move the surgery to a point fifteen hours later. Why?"

Again, a pause. Longer this time, as the question hung in the air, almost visibly. Chris took a deep breath. "Dr. Zide, on Tuesday night my band and I debut at Carnegie Hall."

I took a deep breath, but I knew what I had to do. You'd have done the same. I got back onto the telephone and spent a harrowing forty-five minutes rescheduling the OR time.

The thought never crossed my mind that Chris would play the trombone again, but six months later, after having most of his upper lip muscles removed, he had figured out a way to come close to his original embouchure. He was able to get a few toots out of his beloved trombone.

Six years later, I saw him once for follow-up. He smiled broadly as he handed me his new CD and told me that once more he was leading his band.

Incredible!

JERONIMO

EDMOND A. ZINGARO, M.D.
SAN FRANCISCO, CA

Go for the jugular of mediocrity. To never give up and to never be sat-
isfied with second best depends on dedicated determination through
motivation engendered by pride in perfection.
    −Ralph Millard, M.D.

Surgery in the third world presents a whole set of circumstances very different from those of more advanced countries. What would be a routine procedure in the United
States can become a demanding challenge with a corre-
spondingly greater chance of failure. Since my days as a
plastic surgery resident, I have been involved in traveling
with surgical teams providing service in these dramatically
poorer areas, so I know this from long experience.

Take the case of Jeronimo.

Some twelve years back, I was working in the jungles of
northwestern Guatemala. A man arrived in the clinic, bringing with him a baby who had been born with a unilateral
cleft lip and palate. Nutrition standards being what they are
in that part of the world, children are routinely small, and
this little guy was no different. He was nearly eleven months
old, but looked half that age. Other than his small size, he
appeared to be in decent health. We scheduled a repair of his
cleft lip.

The surgery itself was uneventful; a Millard repair was completed. But by that evening, he was beginning to look sick.
We soon recognized that he had developed all the signs of

sepsis, and it became clear that his body was not winning its fight.

Imagine the scene. We were in a small, under-equipped clinic in the middle of nowhere, trying to figure out how, with our limited resources, we were going to save this little kid. An aggressive sepsis is very bad news, even in a well-equipped American hospital. In a Guatemalan jungle, it was a harbinger of doom.

Improvisation was needed, and quickly. The small recovery area had an air conditioner, so it immediately became the intensive care unit. We broke out all the fancy antibiotics brought from stateside, and worked out the dosages. Someone found an old Bird respirator in the basement. It took a bit of work, but we got it functioning and intubated little Jeronimo to help his breathing.

Yes, Jeronimo was his real name.

Members of our group stayed by his bedside all night – checking vital signs, administering medications, adjusting the respirator, and, in general, watching over him with greatest attention. The team chant became "Jeronimo, Jeronimo, Jeronimo!"

Whether the boy heard and responded to our battle cries, or whether it was the care we were able to give him, we would never know. The fact was that within forty-eight hours he showed signs of improvement. And by the time we were ready to leave the clinic and return to the United States, he was well on the road to recovery and hospital discharge. We ended up calling ourselves on that trip "Team Jeronimo."

Over the next several years, I often took groups back to that clinic. Many of the same doctors, nurses, and other members came with me.

Then, just ten years after the Jeronimo incident, I was back in the same place working with my team. Looking over the clinic's patient list, I noted a patient named "Jeronimo." The events of a decade earlier leapt immediately into sharp focus in my memory. I pulled out the patient's chart and soon found my own handwritten notes, with my signature underneath.

Jeronimo had come back!

His father opened the door to the examination room, bringing his son with him. Jeronimo Senior immediately remembered me and broke into a long discourse about how I was famous in their village for saving his son's life and putting him on the road to recovery.

It was an overwhelming experience. Jeronimo, now ten years old, had developed into a very healthy boy. He had returned to the clinic several times for follow-up procedures before this visit and now had only one minor defect where the cleft palate had been repaired – a small fistula. We operated on him and eliminated the fistula.

With everything now in good shape, he left our care. As he went, we hugged him and his family before bidding them a most heartfelt farewell.

Jeronimo had been a most rewarding patient.

NO INTRODUCTION NECESSARY

HILTON BECKER, M.D.   BOCA RATON, FL

Men govern nothing with more difficulty than their tongues.
–Spinoza

I normally introduce myself to my new consultations. On this particular day, we were having a pretty hectic morning and I rushed in to see the patient.

A new chart was on the door so I put out my hand to introduce myself, stating, "Good morning, I'm Dr. Becker . . .pleased to meet you." The patient turned around and said, "Dr. Becker, I'm Mrs. Jones. You did a facelift on me two weeks ago." My answer to her was, "Well, see how good you look? I didn't even recognize you."

WERE IT NOT FOR YOU

JEFFREY S. ROSENTHAL, M.D.
FAIRFIELD, CT

That life is worth living is the most necessary of assumptions and, were it not assumed, the most impossible of conclusions.
–Santayana

Daniel was seventeen years old when he came close to losing his life.

At an outdoor barbecue party, somebody made the not very clever decision to pour gasoline over the charcoal briquettes to start the fire. Unaware of what was being done, Daniel was so close to the barbecue that the leaping flames engulfed him, setting his clothes alight, and inflicting terrible, life-threatening burns over much of his body.

I first saw him just a few hours later in our hospital, where he had been rushed for vital resuscitation and therapy. He was almost completely covered in bandages from head to toe. Monitors beeped, oxygen was delivered to him through a ventilator, fluids ran through several tubes to sustain his damaged body. Fortunately for him, he was unaware of his perilous situation – he was deeply asleep.

That first visit to Daniel's bedside was the beginning of an eight-year relationship. In those early weeks, it was a difficult and stormy one. It later progressed from those first steps to pull him back from the brink, to the weary and painful procedures of long-term recovery and rehabilitation, and finally to wellness.

After the first few days, Daniel became able to breathe on his own, without mechanical assistance. This was a turning point in his therapy, but it brought with it additional problems in the management of his case. Surgery progressed by stages, with the aim of salvaging and reconstructing his face, ears, lips, eyelids, and neck. It was a unique challenge because such large areas were involved. We had to remove the unhealthy, damaged tissues layer by layer, while at the same time maintaining the underlying healthy structures.

The discomfort that Daniel endured during these early phases of treatment was exacerbated by the fear he felt. The psychological trepidation was often more powerful than the physical pain, and I could only manage it effectively by talking, cajoling, and sometimes by simply insisting that he cooperate. This process was why our relationship was initially such a contentious one.

However, his personality was strong enough to come through these agonies and uncertainties; and in doing so, he became a new person. He still had to undergo many other interventions to reshape and reform the delicate and visible areas of his face; he still had to go through the normal anxieties before and after each operation. But he learned that my prime concern was to work as his surgeon with his best interest always in mind.

Eventually, after his long and hard journey through pain and anxiety, Daniel was released from the hospital. His introduction to physical therapy at our hospital prompted him to assist in therapy at other hospitals and to train for that skill. He went back to ice hockey, his high school sport. His mind and his body continued to grow and mature in a positive way, and he became an outgoing, charming, and productive member of the town's community.

Eight years after his devastating injury, my wife and I got an invitation to Daniel's wedding. We were flattered to be asked and set aside the few hours to attend the celebration of his marriage. To our surprise and delight, we found ourselves to be a center of attention. His friends and close relations treated us as part of his family.

The highlight came when the best man lifted his champagne glass to toast the joyful couple. To my astonishment, his first words were not of congratulations to the newlyweds, but of thanks to me, for making this day possible.

The unseen but very real emotional bond that Daniel and I had forged through many years of interaction – sometimes painful, sometimes difficult, but ultimately rewarding – touched me deeply. That day was truly a celebration of life.

TROUBLED WATERS

NARENDRA PANDYA, M.D. BOMBAY, INDIA

Experience is the name everyone
gives to his mistakes.
–Oscar Wilde

A community just north of Bombay, middle-of-the-road in everything economic, social, educational – has one characteristic which manifests itself in all members: reticence.

These people are unusually self-contained and shy. They keep very much to themselves and are reluctant to discuss their personal problems with anyone, even a professional such as a doctor.

From this background came a young lady of twenty-seven, attractive, married, and the mother of two children. All very normal. But she had a concern, a worry, which came close to taking over her entire life. She had tiny breasts.

A fact of life, you might say, simply part of her physical make-up. And that conclusion would have been true but for the fact her that her small bosom increasingly irritated her husband, who frequently taunted her about it, insisting that she must have something done to correct the situation. In short, she was having serious problems with her marriage. In a more open society than hers, she would have sought a remedy and consulted a plastic surgeon. But her shyness and reserve militated against such an obvious solution. She could not face being seen as having such a consultation. She would become the shamefaced talk of the town.

Bombay is home to a number of surgeons of subprofessional standards – poorly trained and inexperienced, but inexpensive. The lady in question finally resorted to one of these low-level practitioners, having seen one of his many advertisements in the local press. He checked her over, and agreed to carry out a procedure to augment her breasts. The fee would be relatively small, and none of her acquaintances would be any the wiser.

She went along with his proposal and chose a date when her husband would be away on business. The back-street doctor operated, putting in saline-filled implants as a bilateral augmentation. Surprisingly, the surgery went well. No infections, no adverse after-effects other than several days of discomfort. Soon she was able to return home.

After two or three weeks, her husband was back with her, and they resumed their lovemaking. Things did not go well, however, because whenever they were moving vigorously in the course of sex, they were disturbed with the sound of splashing water emanating from her breasts.

He became more and more upset by this interference with their intimacy and eventually became as angry as he had been about the smallness of her breasts. She had not told him about the mammoplasty – she had kept it a secret from him as much as she had from her friends – so he was as perplexed as he was angry. After a month or so, he was so furious that he refused to be with her at night. The marriage was again becoming a wreck.

She went back to her fly-by-night surgeon and explained her problem. He insisted that he had made no mistakes in the procedure, that the problem was in some way of her own making.

By now she was desperate. Throwing aside her natural reserve, she came to see me and related the story of her past miserable three months. From her description of the symptoms, it was obvious that air had somehow found its way into the saline bags while the liquid was being infiltrated.

I persuaded her to let me replace the implants and to avoid any recurrence of this distressing situation. Surgery and recovery were both without problems, the marriage was repaired, and the lady – still shy, still reserved, took up a happier way of life.

When I talk about this with my colleagues, they are amused by envisaging the night-time scenes between husband and wife. They don't fully realize the suffering the lady went through because of the actions of an incompetent surgeon.

TOUCHED BY A HAND

STEVEN HOFFLIN, M.D.
SANTA MONICA, CA

Simple pleasures . . . are the last
refuge of the complex.
–Wilde

In 1976, I was the lead surgeon in replanting an amputated hand in surgery performed at UCLA Harbor General Hospital, with the plastic surgical team and Chief of Service, Malcolm Lessavoy, M.D.

A young male in his 20s had been driving with his left hand out of the window. The car rolled over, amputating the hand. In an hours-long procedure, we successfully replanted it.

For many years, I received cards and thank-yous from this patient. There was one which was especially touching to me that was written by his replanted hand. I understood that he was able to strum a guitar and lead a reasonably productive life. This is what makes medicine so satisfying to all of us.

PUBIC MOUSTACHE

VACLAV POLACEK, PH.D.
PRAGUE CZECH REPUBLIC

I must complain the cards are ill-shuffled,
till I have a good hand.
–Swift

This story is approximately 15 years old and it happened when the Czech Republic and Slovakia were one state – Czechoslovakia.

Under the communist regime, it was the rule that young men spent their military service far from home. That meant Czechs in Slovakia and Slovaks in Bohemia.

At the time, I was working at the burn division of the plastic surgery department of Charles University in Prague. A young Slovak soldier was brought in. He had third-degree burns all over his body, the worst of which were on his head and around his lips. During his stay in the hospital, he told someone he had a girl; after his tour of duty was over they were supposed to get married. His mother came to the hospital to offer support. I took her aside to explain her son's disfigurement and also to warn her that the girl her son had been dating might break the engagement. The soldier's mother shook her head saying, "This is a well-behaved girl. She will not go back on her word." The soldier was sent home and he and his fiance announced the date of their wedding.

At the next check-up, the patient came with his father, who asked me, "You know, Doctor, in our village we are accustomed to men in moustaches. And we wish one for our son. Can you please make him a moustache?" I felt uneasy. Hair transplantation was at its beginning. The patient had burn scars on his head, so the only hair without defect would have to come from the genitals. The decision was to reconstruct the upper lip, using a large, full thickness skin graft containing skin follicles from the pubic area. I was very surprised at how well the transplant healed and how soon hair started to grow.

Several months later, the patient came in for a visit and showed us his wedding photographs. He proudly pointed out his moustache. After he left, the nurses asked if we noticed that strange moustache? I explained its origin. One nurse blurted out, "I'm glad I didn't kiss him."

I received a demijohn of plum brandy made in 1983 from this soldier. It is still in our pantry; it reminds me of the year of that surgery.

Chapter X
Self-Reliance

CHAPTER OF ACCIDENTS

STEPHAN ARIYAN, M.D.   NEW HAVEN, CT

To measure up to what is demanded of him, a man
must overestimate his capacities.
–Goethe

Elizabeth is a psychotherapist who came to see me about a facelift. Aged 68, she had lost her husband six years earlier. More recently she had retired from the university where she was on the faculty and moved into an old house with a barn in the northern part of Vermont, a five-hour drive away from my office. She had made that long trip for the consultation and planned to return home that afternoon and telephone to let us know if she had decided to go ahead with the procedure.

All this I knew about her. What I didn't know was that she would turn out to be the most determined patient I ever came across in my practice.

My office is in a large medical tower building, with an attached indoor multi-level garage. After the consultation, on her way from the lobby to the elevators which would take her to the parking area, she tripped and fell. The lobby security guard saw her fall and went to her aid. As she regained her feet and dusted herself off he couldn't help noticing that she showed signs of quite severe tenderness of the wrist.

He felt that she should come back to see me, but she refused, telling him that there was a long drive ahead of her, and she wanted to get back home before dark. She went on down to the garage, found her car, and drove away. The guard came to tell me what had happened and voiced his concern that

274

she had possibly injured her wrist.

I called her later that evening to check that she had arrived home safely and that there was no problem with the wrist. Her reply was that she felt that the wrist had in fact been broken by the fall but had decided to drive home before seeking treatment. To have waited for the application of a cast would have meant a late-night return, and this she did not want.

She added that her ankle had also given her trouble during the drive and that when she arrived in Burlington, she went immediately to her orthepedic surgeon. He told her that not only was her wrist broken, but her ankle was broken as well. She ended the call by postponing any plans for the face-lift until after her recovery.

* * * * * * *

A year went by. Her fractures completely healed, Elizabeth came back to my office for further consultation. She was determined to proceed with the facelift, so I made the arrangements.

The operation went smoothly. She recovered for a few days at a medical accommodation facility connected to the office building – convenient, as it allows for the patient to relax in a hotel environment while at the same time being under the direct supervision of nurses and healthcare providers.

On the fourth postoperative day, she came back to my office. The dressings and fine sutures around the eyelids and in front of the ear were removed. Before she left, I explained that I'd need to see her in another week to remove the staples within the scalp and in the back of the ear.

She wanted to drive back to Vermont that afternoon; I felt that she was doing well enough to be able to drive. Then she took me by surprise. She could not, she said, return a week later because it was Vermont's rainy season. Once the rains came, the dirt road which served as her driveway would be impassable.

I recovered from speechlessness. "But what will you do about groceries and other supplies?"

"Oh, I've already stocked the place up, as I always do in the spring rainy season."

I had not planned on this turn of events when scheduling the operation. Elizabeth, though, was working to her own agenda. It was only with a lot of reluctance that she called me to make arrangements for the Visiting Nurse Association to check on her at home – travel conditions permitting! – and to remove the staples for her.

The very next day, I got a call from the Association to tell me that she would not let them come to see her. I called her back at once. She insisted that she was doing very well, that she would take care of the staples, and that she had no need to see a physician at that stage.

Another dramatic turn came a week later. A nurse from the the VNA telephoned to tell me that she had received an urgent call from Elizabeth, asking her to come out to her home to see her. Apparently she had gone to the barn to take down a thirty-pound roll of baling wire from a top shelf. She lost her grip on the wire, which fell and struck her on the left side of her face.

When the nurse arrived, she saw that Elizabeth's face was heavily bruised, swollen, and discolored black and blue. Even so, she refused to go to the emergency room. She just wanted the nurse to check that the face-lift operation had not been damaged. With another display of her usual reluctance, she finally agreed to go to see a plastic surgeon near her home.

This surgeon was quite clearly amazed by the story as it unfolded. After he had examined my patient, he called to tell us that, apart from soft-tissue swelling and the black and blue discoloration, everything was OK.

As I said at the beginning, Elizabeth was the most self-reliant and determined patient I've ever come across in my professional career.

And, let me add, the one who caused me the greatest anguish.

THE LONG HAUL

STEPHAN ARIYAN, M.D.
NEW HAVEN, CT

*At least be sure that you go to the author
to get at his meaning, not to find yours.*
–Ruskin

Anita was young, healthy, bubbling with energy, and quite unstoppable. But she had a severe and debilitating problem – very large and heavy breasts, which caused her much pain and discomfort of the neck and shoulders. In search of help, she came to see me. After consultation and examination, I decided that she was a good candidate for a reduction mammoplasty.

The operation was carried out without incident, and she was in my Connecticut office on a Thursday, two days later, for follow-up examination. She had made a rapid recuperation, and so when she asked if it would be all right for her to visit her sister in Washington for the weekend, I immediately agreed. There could be no harm in her taking the train to Washington, D.C. for a brief visit and then returning.

Two days later, my answering service reported that she had called me. I returned the call. She told me that she was experiencing significant pain in both breasts. Being unsure whether she had followed through on her travel plans, I asked where she was calling from.

"Chicago," she replied.

It took me no time at all to realize that I had made the mistake of assuming that she had planned to go to Washington, D.C., when in fact her sister lived in Washington state – Seattle, as it turned out, on the far northwest coast.

"Are you calling from O'Hare airport?" I asked her.

"No, I'm at a gas station."

"What are you doing there?"

"Oh, I'm just filling up my tank – it's a long drive to Seattle!"

Two misunderstandings, then. Different destination, different schedule – her plans were not for a weekend, but for a week.

I was able to call on a medical facility to help her alleviate the pain she was suffering, but the episode taught me to adopt a much more questioning attitude when sanctioning patients' requests to go ahead with postoperative activities.

SLUGGER

MARJORIE CRAMER, M.D.   BROOKLYN, NY

For violence, like Achilles' lance,
can heal the wounds it has inflicted.
    –Frantz Fanon

My first really funny moment occurred when I was doing the General Surgery part of the residency. I worked very hard, was technically good, and I managed to get on well with the other residents. One day my chief resident asked me, with a twinkle in his eye, if men followed me when I walked down the street. After a few moments of watching my amazed reaction, he explained that the evaluation form that Dr. Dennis asked the chief residents to fill out about the residents had the question "is he a leader of men?" I never did ask him how he filled mine out.

In my intern year, most of the complement of interns was drafted to serve in the Vietnam War and we were disastrously understaffed and overworked, even for interns. I had the great distinction of being the only intern, however, who worked two straight months on the trauma service without backup, meaning that I was up all night every other night. There was much too much work to do, and I was constantly running from OR to ER to ward, and was chronically tired and cranky.

One morning at 8 a.m., after spending the better part of the night in the OR, I heard a page to the ER as I peeled off my gloves. I immediately went to the ER and to my surprise found that the admitting surgery resident was extremely angry with me, saying that he had been paging me for over an hour and intimated that I had been avoiding my page, presumably by oversleeping. I began to explain that I had not heard the page in the OR but his angry face glowering redly at me just made something snap; before I knew what I was doing, I slapped him hard. He stepped back in amazement, removed his eyeglasses and carefully put them in his pocket. I presume this was a first for him.

Later, I was very upset and called my long-suffering and wonderfully supportive husband and told him that I was afraid I would get fired. Well, I didn't, but it seems that after that incident people treated me with more respect, so the story has a happy ending and I have a few friends who still call me "slugger!"

EULOGY FOR MICHAEL L. LEWIN, M.D.

BERISH STRAUCH, M.D.   BRONX, NY

A good reputation is more valuable than money.
–Publilius Syrus, approximately 100 B.C.

This following was presented at Dr. Lewin's funeral services, May 12, 1997:

How does one measure the accomplishment of an individual whose span and deeds had such enormous impact on so many people? Recounting Michael's professional benchmarks of starting and directing the Plastic Surgery Service at Montefiore Hospital in 1958; initiating the combined Albert Einstein/Montefiore Medical Center program in 1976; remaining as Director of the Weiler service for the past ten years; starting, developing, and nurturing the international scenes in plastic surgery – all of these do not really tell us in any accurate way what this unusual person was like.

Michael Lewin, the plastic surgeon, will be remembered literally by thousands of patients and the families of these patients, whom he cared for with his hands, mind, and heart. He touched their lives, and they were better for it. The young baby who lost his nose was cared for with warmth, kindness, and brilliance, through all the many years of surgical intervention. Today, wherever that young man is, he will remember.

Michael Lewin, the teacher, will be remembered by many medical students and over 80 plastic surgery residents whom he has trained and whose lives he has touched. Many of them are here in the audience today. Michael had a unique and incisive method of Socratic teaching which caused students to give more of themselves than even they knew they were capable of. Michael Lewin, the Professor of Plastic Surgery, leaves a legacy to all of us among the outstanding group of plastic surgeons he has trained. These trainees are now practicing throughout this country and around the world, caring for their own patients. They will remember.

Michael Lewin, as colleague and faculty member, will remain in the memories of all his associates – surgeons, nurses, and administrators – as a visionary with plans to have the best plastic surgery services, giving his own almost inexhaustible energy to this task. In his middle sixties, when many are contemplating easing off a bit, he traveled to France to work with a similar soul, in learning and developing a whole new specialty: craniofacial surgery. He brought these skills back to the Bronx. His legacy of scientific articles continues to influence the plastic surgery community to this day. For all of his contributions to the Department, to the faculty, and to the plastic surgery community, he will be remembered.

Michael, as a personal friend, mentor, and colleague, will always remain close to me in my thoughts and in my heart. When I was a young general surgical resident, he took me under his wing and invited my wife and me to his home, where I first met Berta and the children. His sage advice and help led me, early on in my training, to the specialty of hand surgery, and then to plastic surgery. I came back to New York to work with Michael (Dr. Lewin at the time) in 1968.

Our professional relationship continued, matured, and even

changed roles; but the respect and love we both had for each other never changed. One of the hardest things that I ever had to do was after Michael's 80th birthday: I asked him to stop operating, and he reluctantly agreed. He was an amazing person: He would operate all day and then, when other people went home exhausted, he would go home and swim a couple of miles, and play singles tennis. Although he agreed to stop operating in the operating room, he asked me if he could continue to operate and do some surgery in the office. When I asked him what kind of office procedures he planned to do, he said sheepishly, "a facelift or maybe a rhinoplasty." He continued to provide advice, guidance, and support, even into the time of his illness. For all of this, I will remember.

To Berta. You have always been at his side, supporting him, helping him to develop his ideas and the realization of those ideas, and supporting the family in ways that wives of visionaries and committed men need. He knew, and he will always remember.